Clinical Dermatology

Dr Neil H Cox
Consultant Dermatologist
Cumberland Infirmary
Carlisle, UK

Dr Clifford M Lawrence
Consultant Dermatologist
Royal Victoria Infirmary
Newcastle, UK

M Mosby

London   Baltimore   Bogotá   Boston   Buenos Aires   Caracas   Carlsbad, CA   Chicago   Madrid   Mexico City
Milan   Naples, FL   New York   Philadelphia   St. Louis   Sydney   Tokyo   Toronto   Wiesbaden

Project Manager:	Jane Hurd-Cosgrave
Developmental Editor:	Jennifer Prast
Production:	Joe Lynch
Index:	Anita Reid
Publisher:	Richard Furn

MOSBY
An imprint of Harcourt Publishers Limited

M is a registered trademark of Harcourt Publishers Limited

First published in 1995 by Mosby-Wolfe
  Reprinted 1999

ISBN 0 7234 2193 5

British Library Cataloguing in Publication Data
A catalogue record for this book is available from the British Library.

Library of Congress Cataloging in Publication Data
A catalog record for this book is available from the Library of Congress.

Printed in China
GCC/02

Preface

Diagnostic Picture Tests in Clinical Dermatology is written primarily as a self-test for readers preparing for general practice or general medical postgraduate examinations. Medical students, physicians and general practitioners can also use it to update their dermatology expertise, since the answers are sufficiently detailed to teach as well as to test. We have tried to produce questions which are not simply a test of recognition; where there is a learning component in either the pathway to a diagnosis or an important aspect of investigation or therapy, this has been emphasized in the answer. Common conditions are well represented, particularly if the correct diagnosis has important management implications. Dermatological manifestations of systemic disease are also prominently included, as these are of importance to non-dermatologists.

Acknowledgements

We are grateful to our families for their support during preparation of this book. A small number of illustrations have been used previously by the authors in articles in *Pulse* and *Update*, and a few in *Physical Signs in Dermatology* (Mosby–Year Book Europe 1993) by the same authors.

1 ▶

This man suddenly developed a widespread rash, with weepy, crusted areas on his head and neck.

a. What features are shown?

b. What is the differential diagnosis?

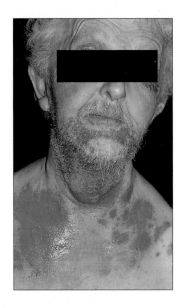

2 ▶

This acute eruption on the sole of the foot was triggered by a recent infection.

a. What is the eponymous name of this condition?

b. What was the likely site of the associated infection?

c. What other symptoms may occur?

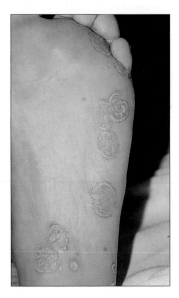

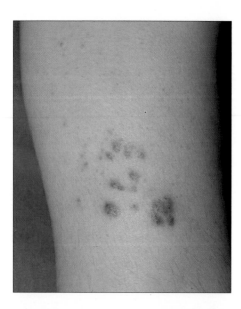

◀ 3

This young woman had several areas of grouped, bluish, compressible, non-painful nodules arising on her trunk and limbs. Her father had similar lesions.

a. What is the differential diagnosis?

b. With what may they be confused if thrombosis occurs?

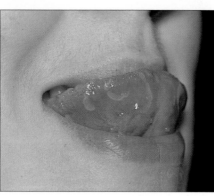

◀ 4

This patient has variable lesions on the tongue.

a. What is the name of this condition?

b. What is the usual significance?

c. In which dermatoses may similar changes occur?

5 ▶

The nodule shown here had enlarged steadily over several years. A foul-smelling, cheesy material was present when the cyst was incised.

a. What is the diagnosis?
b. What are the contents?

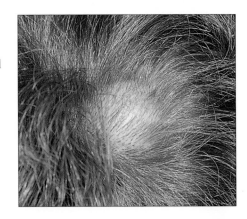

6 ▶

This patient was referred to the clinic with 'bruising' of the penis.

a. What is the likely diagnosis?
b. Why does pur-pura occur?
c. What symptoms may be present?

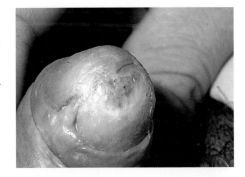

7 ▶

The child in this illustration had been treated for scabies two months earlier, but still had itchy papules in his axillae and groins.

a. What is the diagnosis?
b. Is further scabies treatment needed?

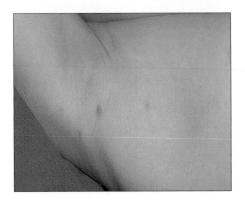

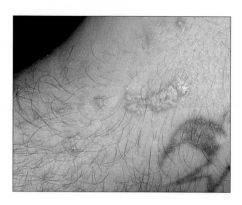

◀ 8

The illustration shows an itchy rash on the arm of a male patient.
a. What is the likely diagnosis?
b. What two eponymous features of the disorder are illustrated here?
c. How would you use a torch to strengthen your diagnosis?

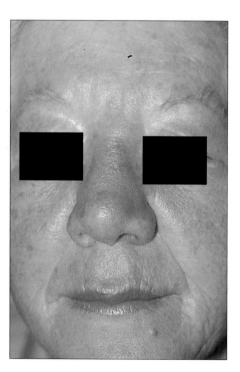

◀ 9

This patient suffers with swelling and tenderness of the face, of acute onset.
a. What is the differential diagnosis?
b. What investigations would you perform?

10 ▶

These lesions have developed on the tongue of a young male patient.

a. Give two possible diagnoses.

b. This man had purplish nodules on the legs and palate; what condition do the findings suggest?

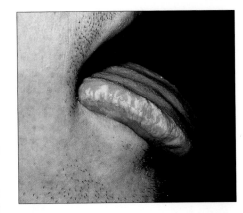

11 ▶

This child had an itchy rash after a holiday.

a. What is the diagnosis?

b. What is the possible cause?

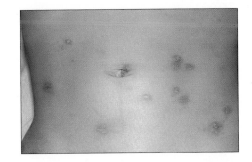

12 ▶

In the condition shown, skin lesions frequently occur over over bony prominences.

a. How would you describe the illustrated lesions?

b. What is the likely diagnosis?

c. What skeletal feature is likely?

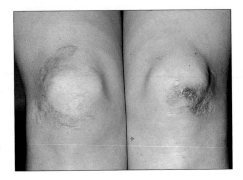

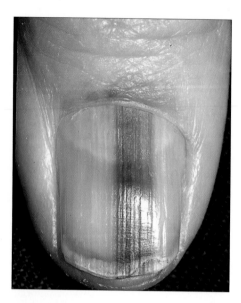

◀ 13
The black streak shown here has slowly developed in the fingernail of an elderly woman.
a. What other feature is shown?
b. What is the likely diagnosis?
c. How would you confirm the diagnosis?

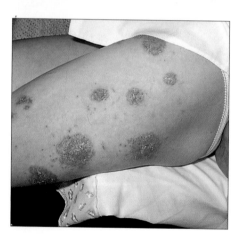

◀ 14
The illustration shows an intensely itchy rash, of acute onset.
a. Describe the lesions shown.
b. What is the likely diagnosis?
c. How would you treat the condition?

15 ▶

This patient had applied topical steroids for what was presumed to be foot eczema, but the rash became worse.

a. What physical signs are present?

b. What is the cause?

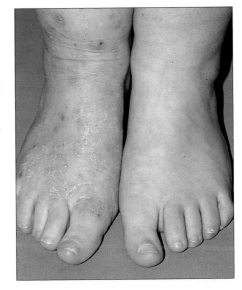

16 ▶

These are important physical signs presented by a patient to demonstrate the cause of her pruritus.

a. What is the likely diagnosis?

b. What test should be performed?

c. Which drug is usually used for this condition?

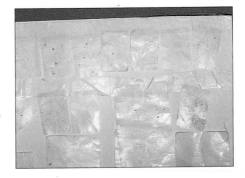

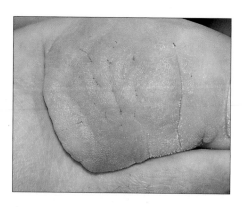

◀ 17

This patient was referred from the general medical clinic with diffuse non-pitting swelling of her shins and feet.

a. What feature is shown on the top of her great toe?

b. What is the cause?

c. What nail abnormality may be associated?

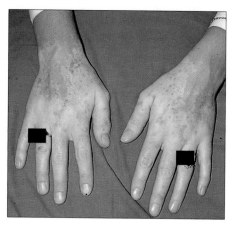

◀ 18

This patient presented with skin colour change on the hands.

a. What is the likely diagnosis?

b. What further investigations may be carried out?

c. To which of the colours should the patient apply a sunscreen?

19 ▶

A young woman reported that a mole, which had been present for years, had started to change.
a. What is the probable diagnosis?
b. How should this be managed?

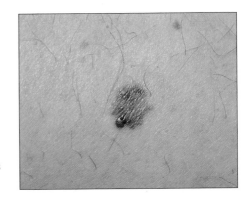

20 ▶

This patient reported an itchy lesion on the sole of the foot, after a foreign holiday.
a. Describe the features shown.
b. What is the likely diagnosis?
c. What infestation usually causes this?

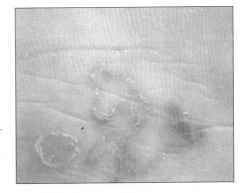

21 ▶

The woman in this illustration has had three transient ischaemic attacks.
a. How would you describe the skin abnormality on her legs?
b. Can you relate this to the cerebral ischaemia?

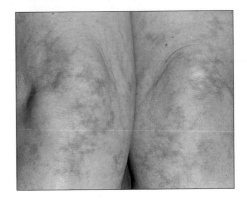

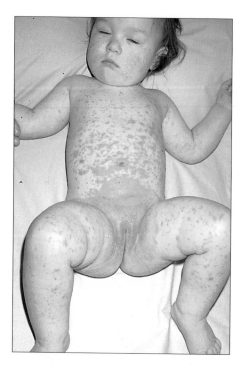

◀ 22
This infant has an extensive rash which is essentially asymptomatic.
a. What is the likely diagnosis?
b. What scalp change may be present?
c. What is the prognosis?

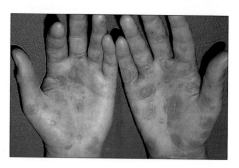

◀ 23
This patient has developed recurrent crops of blisters.
a. What feature is shown?
b. What is the most likely diagnosis?
c. What are the possible causes?

24 ▶

The illustration shows a plaque behind the ear of an elderly man.

a. What are the two most likely diagnoses?

b. What question may help in the differential diagnosis?

c. What test may be required?

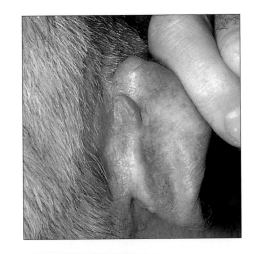

25 ▶

A patient became pyrexial and rapidly developed wide-spread red scaling areas with peripheral pustules.

a. Give two likely diagnoses.

b. How would you manage the most likely one?

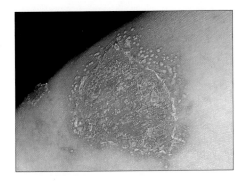

26 ▶

This asymptomatic rash has occurred on the abdomen of an elderly widower.

a. What abnormal findings are illustrated?

b. What is the likely diagnosis?

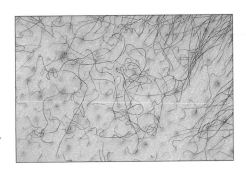

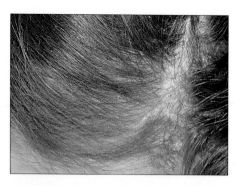

◄ 27
There is severe scaling and itching on the scalp of this child.
a. What is the probable diagnosis?
b. What other features would you look for?

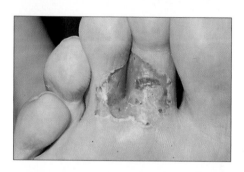

◄ 28
This patient complains of an itchy rash on the foot.
a. What is the likely diagnosis?
b. What test might be helpful?

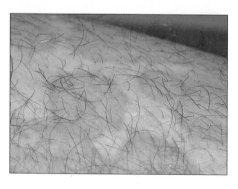

◄ 29
This man had itchy, red plaques on the trunk and limbs. Individual lesions resolved spontaneously within 24 hours, and new ones subsequently appeared.
a. What is the diagnosis?
b. What investigations are required?

30 ▶

The eyelid lesions shown here were an incidental finding in this young girl with a respiratory illness.

a. What abnormality is shown?

b. What is the likely cause?

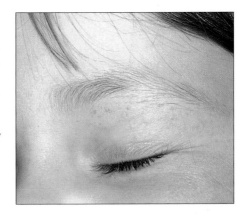

31 ▶

This woman developed a rash and patchy hair loss.

a. What features are seen in this close-up view?

b. What is the probable diagnosis?

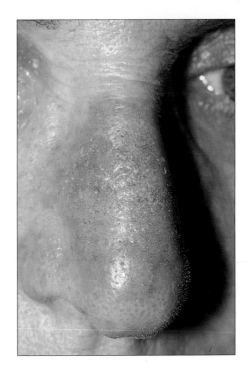

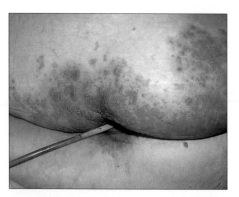

◀ **32**

This woman suffers from a painful eruption on the buttock.

a. What is the diagnosis?
b. Why is a urinary catheter *in situ*?
c. What other complications may occur at this site?

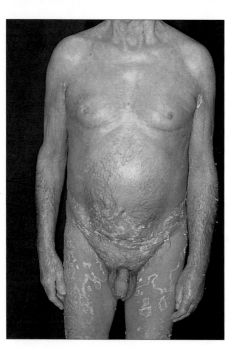

◀ **33**

This man developed the widespread rash shown here over a period of 10 days.

a. How would you describe the rash?
b. Give four possible causes.
c. List potential immediate complications.

34 ▶

This child has been brought to the clinic with a popliteal rash.
a. What is the likely diagnosis?
b. Name four cardinal clinical features of this disorder.
c. What viral infection can be dangerous in patients with this condition?

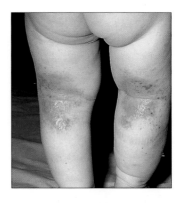

35 ▶

This is a close-up view of the edge of a bald area in a man with patchy hair loss.
a. What abnormality is shown?
b. What is the diagnosis?
c. What other features would you look for?

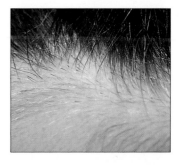

36 ▶

An elderly man presents with these lesions on his trunk.
a. What is the name of these common lesions?
b. The patient had a large number of the lesions, of many years duration. Does this have any important significance?

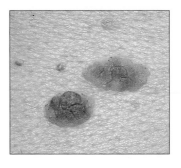

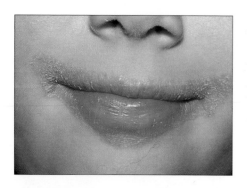

◄ 37

The child in this illustration attended the clinic with a perioral rash.

a. Describe the features shown.

b. What is the differential diagnosis?

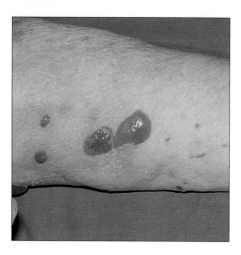

◄ 38

These blisters were seen on the upper arm of an elderly woman.

a. Describe the salient features illustrated which are of diagnostic importance.

b. The blisters were preceded by eczematous patches. There was no mucosal involvement. What is the likely diagnosis?

c. What investigation should be performed?

39 ▶

This child has developed these asymptomatic lesions of the chin.

a. What is the likely diagnosis?

b. What is the prognosis?

c. How would you treat the lesions?

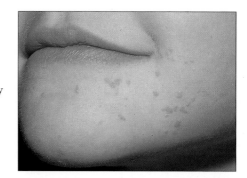

40 ▶

This elderly patient had a painless ulcer on the sole of her foot, and haemorrhagic blisters on the tips of her toes.

a. What process is the cause of these changes?

b. What may be the underlying disease?

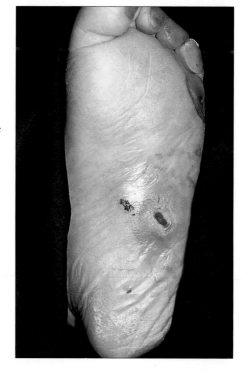

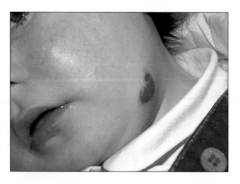

◀ 41

This child was born with a red nodule on her cheek.

a. What is the diagnosis?

b. What is the prognosis?

c. What are the indications for treatment?

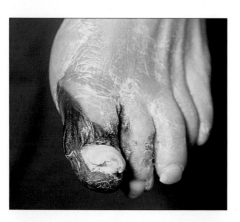

◀ 42

This medical patient presented with an acutely discoloured toe.

a. What is this condition?

b. Apart from arterial disease, what is the likely underlying medical condition?

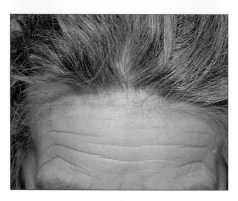

◀ 43

This woman has noticed hair thinning on the front of her scalp.

a. What is striking about the pattern of hair loss?

b. What is the cause?

c. What is the prognosis?

The illustration shows yellowish papules arising on the antihelix of this man's ear.

a. Give three differential diagnoses.

b. What rheumatological feature may help to distinguish between the diagnoses?

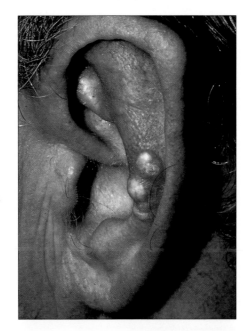

This mother gave birth to a baby with two scalp ulcers. The mother had been born with the same problem, and was left with these two bald areas. At the time, the ulcers had been blamed erroneously on the method of delivery.

a. What abnormality is seen?

b. What is the diagnosis?

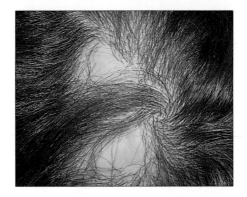

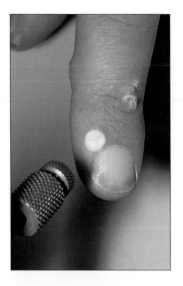

◀ 46

This young man attended the clinic for treatment of the lesions on his fingers.

a. What procedure is being performed here?

b. What is the inevitable side-effect of this treatment?

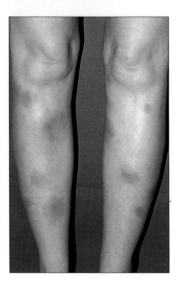

◀ 47

The young woman shown here developed painful nodules on her shins.

a. What is the diagnosis?

b. What possible causes should be considered?

48 ▶

This patient suffers from eyelid lesions.

a. What is the name of these lesions?

b. What serological abnormality will be demonstrated?

c. What is the likely cause of several premature deaths in this patient's family?

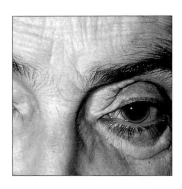

49 ▶

The illustration shows an example of discoloured tongue.

a. What is the diagnosis?

b. Why does this occur?

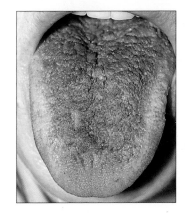

50 ▶

This is a firm, asymptomatic, long-standing lesion on the arm.

a. What is the likely diagnosis?

b. What is the cause of lesions of this type?

c. What is the risk of malignancy if untreated?

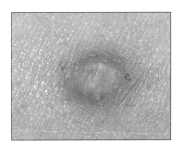

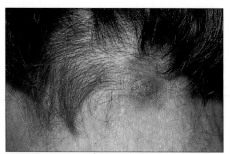

◄ 51
This man has an inflamed nodule on his neck.
a. What is the diagnosis?
b. Are there any predisposing factors?

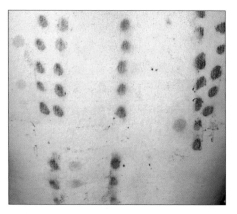

◄ 52
This patient is suffering from a vulval dermatosis.
a. What abnormalities are illustrated?
b. What symptoms are likely?
c. What is the diagnosis?

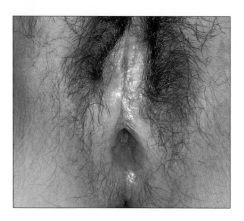

◄ 53
This illustration shows an example of dermatological investigation.
a. What test has been carried out?
b. What skin diseases can be investigated in this way?
c. Why are the ink marks applied?

54 ▶

This male patient, with lesions of the buccal mucosa, also has an itchy skin eruption.

a. What is the likely diagnosis?
b. What proportion of patients have visible oral lesions?
c. What symptoms do the oral lesions usually cause?

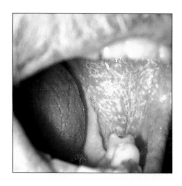

55 ▶

This young man complained of facial and neck flushing.

a. What are the possible causes?

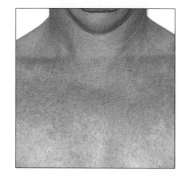

56 ▶

This boy, admitted to hospital as an emergency, displayed the skin lesion shown here.

a. What diagnosis must be considered and treated?
b. What advice would you give his family?

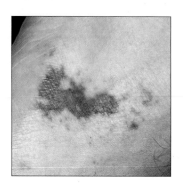

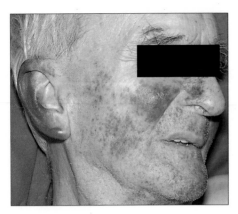

◄ 57

This man became cold and unwell whilst travelling in an aeroplane. He developed wide-spread purpuric areas on his head and neck, hands and feet.

a. What is the striking feature of the distribution?

b. What does this suggest as a likely cause?

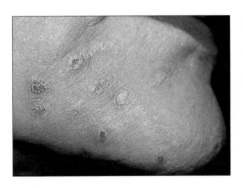

◄ 58

This middle-aged woman suffers from chronic but variable crusted lesions on her chin and cheeks.

a. What is the likely diagnosis?

b. What associated disorder may be present?

c. What is the prognosis?

59 ▶

Small white patches developed on the trunk of this female patient.

a. What features are visible in this close-up view?

b. What is the probable diagnosis?

c. Where else might the patient have signs?

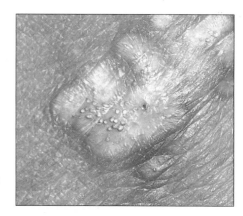

60 ▶

This man, with a previous history of otitis externa, now complains of an itchy rash.

a. What is the likely cause of the new rash?

b. What specific agents may be implicated?

c. What investigation should be performed?

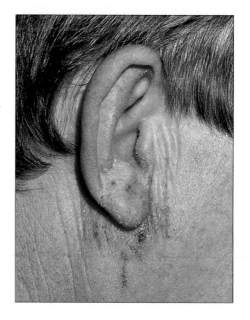

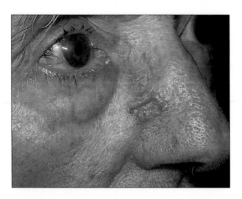

◀ 61
This woman has a slowly growing nodular lesion on the side of her nose.
a. What features are shown?
b. What is the probable diagnosis?
c. What treatment is available?

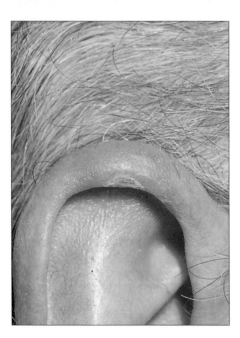

◀ 62
This patient reports a painful nodule of the ear.
a. What is the precise site of the lesion, and why is this important?
b. What is the likely diagnosis?

63 ▶

This female patient, a native of India, has developed a swelling of her foot and discharging sinus.

a. What is the probable diagnosis?

b. What is the likely cause?

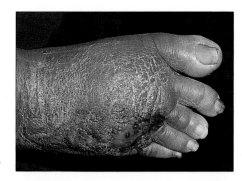

64 ▶

The plant shown in this illustration is the cause of some of the most severe examples of external contact phototoxicity in the UK.

a. What is it?

b. Where is it found?

c. What is the relationship between this plant and the treatment of psoriasis?

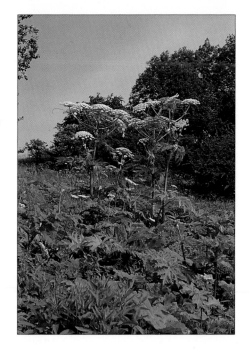

◄ 65
This man had a widespread skin disease. The appearance shown in the illustration was found where he had scratched his back.
a. What is the feature seen?
b. In what disorders does this occur?

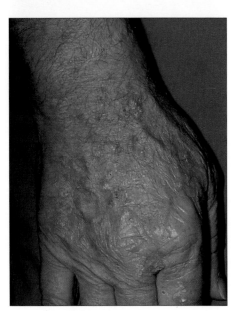

◄ 66
This patient has lesions on the dorsal surface of each hand.
a. Describe the features illustrated.
b. What is the likely diagnosis?
c. Where else might these lesions occur?

67 ▶

This baby was brought to the clinic with large, warty tumours of the perianal skin.

a. What is the diagnosis?

b. What other investigations may be required?

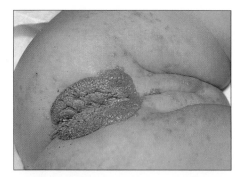

68 ▶

The nail shown here has displayed this abnormality for three months.

a. What is the cause of the discoloration?

b. Is this the cause of the onycholysis?

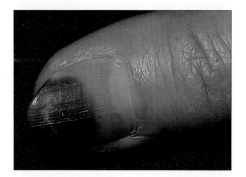

69 ▶

This female patient gradually developed these lesions on her shins.

a. Describe the features shown.

b. What is the diagnosis?

c. What systemic associations are there?

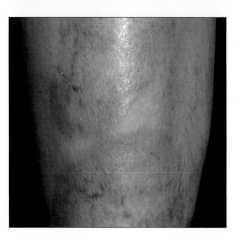

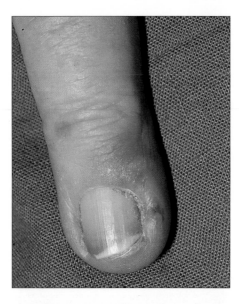

This patient complains of a tender lateral nail-fold. There was no preceding trauma.

a. What is the name of this condition?

b. What organisms may be implicated?

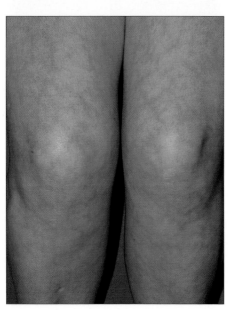

◄ 71

This young woman is concerned about the appearance of the skin on her legs, which, she said, was worse in the cold.

a. What feature is shown?

b. Is investigation required?

72 ▶

This asymptomatic non-scaling lesion on the hand has persisted for six months.

a. What is the likely diagnosis?
b. Why is this unlikely to be a fungal infection?
c. What investigation should be performed?

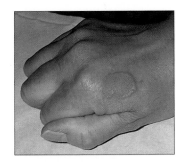

73 ▶

This elderly woman had a long history of pruritus vulvae and, more recently, had noticed a small nodule developing on her vulva.

a. What is the likely diagnosis?
b. What condition may predispose to this?

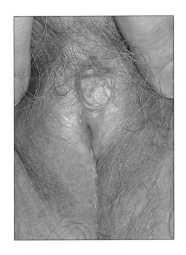

74 ▶

This patient presented with long-standing pigmentation of the penis. The condition illustrated is not due to an abnormality of melanocytes.

a. What is the likely diagnosis?
b. What clinical history would be typical?
c. What agents may be implicated?

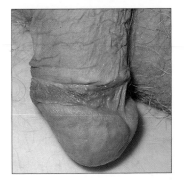

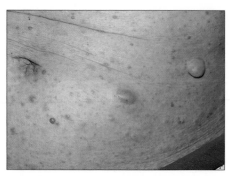

◀ 75

This patient had long-standing soft nodules on the trunk.
a. What is the likely diagnosis?
b. What is the inheritance?
c. What bony complications may occur?

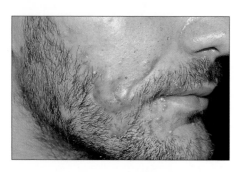

◀ 76

This man has severe scarring on his cheeks and chin.
a. What is this abnormality?
b. How would you treat it?

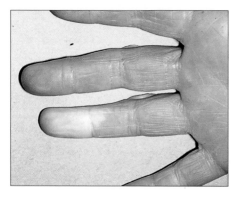

◀ 77

The patient in this case complains of episodic digital colour change with associated pain.
a. What is the likely diagnosis?
b. What are the causes of this condition?
c. Which of the causes is a specific occupational disease?

78 ▶

This woman complained of a brownish, crusted rash under her breasts. Her fingernails showed white streaks and splits. Her father, and his mother, were both believed to have had skin problems.

a. What is the probable diagnosis?
b. What other features would you look for?

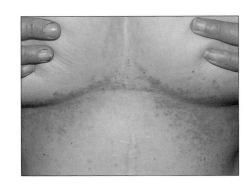

79 ▶

This child suffers from an intensely itchy perianal eruption.

a. What is the likely diagnosis?
b. How would you treat this?
c. A rapidly spreading erythema develops on the child's buttocks; what is the likely explanation?

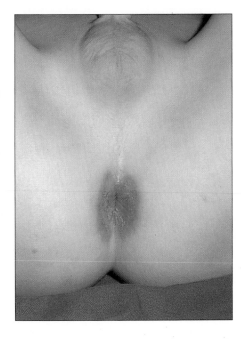

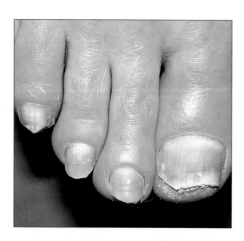

◀ 80
This patient suffers from dystrophic nails.
a. Give two possible causes.
b. Which of these causes is the most likely?
c. How would you confirm this?
d. What treatment is appropriate?

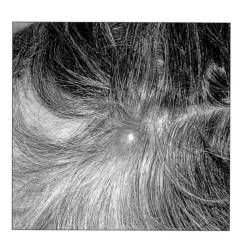

◀ 81
These nodules are found in the scalp of a 65-year-old man with cough and dyspnoea.
a. Why are these not pilar cysts?
b. What diagnosis must be considered?
c. What initial investigations would you perform?

82 ▶

This elderly man presented with slowly increasing, purplish, ill-defined plaques on his feet, head and neck.

a. The plaques are a vascular tumour; what is the likely diagnosis?

b. Serological tests are normal; does this affect your diagnosis?

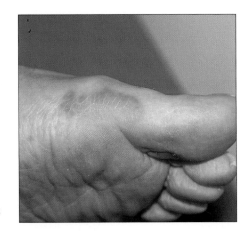

83 ▶

The illustration shows itchy brown spots on the trunk of this child, which become red after rubbing.

a. What is the likely diagnosis?

b. Why do the lesions become red, and what is this sign called?

c. What is the prognosis?

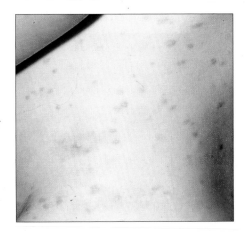

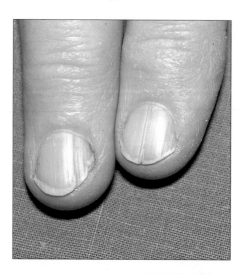

◄ 84
The nail dystrophy shown here is of long-standing.
a. What two abnormalities can be seen?
b. This patient and her mother also had a rash on the trunk. What is the probable diagnosis?
c. What physical sign may be present on the patient's hands?

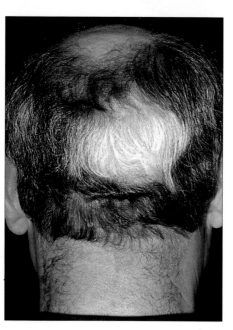

◄ 85
This patient has a history of recent hair loss.
a. What is the likely diagnosis?
b. Would you expect to find white patches of skin elsewhere?

86 ▶

This a close-up view of a newborn baby's skin.

a. What is the cause of the tiny yellow dots?

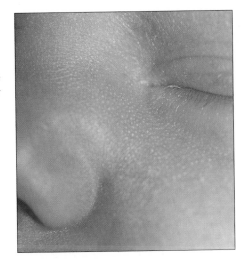

87 ▶

The illustration shows a mildly itchy eruption on the back of a young man.

a. What is the likely diagnosis?

b. How could you prove the diagnosis?

c. What should you warn the patient about when prescribing treatment?

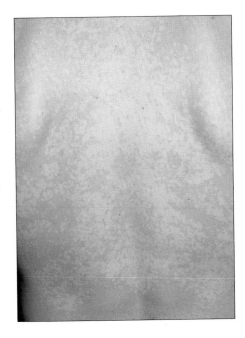

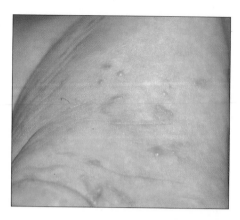

◀ 88

Both this one-year-old child's brother and sister had an itchy rash.
a. What abnormality is present?
b. What is the probable diagnosis?
c. How would you confirm the diagnosis?

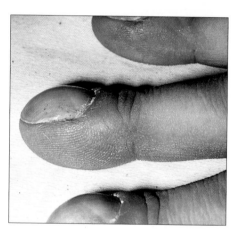

◀ 89

These are the fingers of a 20-year-old patient with chronic medical problems.
a. What two abnormalities are illustrated?
b. What is the likely underlying cause of these two physical signs?
c. What are the other causes of the nail abnormality?

90 ▶

This young girl's toe nails are thickened and grow sideways into the lateral nail fold.

a. What are the possible causes?

b. Which cause is the most likely in this age group?

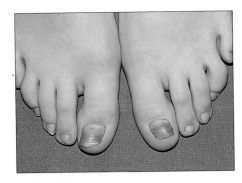

91 ▶

Colour change around a naevus is demonstrated in this illustration.

a. What is the likely diagnosis?

b. Which body site is likely to be affected?

c. The patient is going on holiday; what should you warn him about?

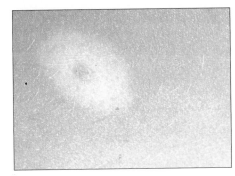

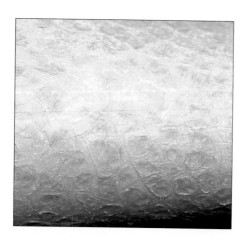

This young man
had suffered from
'dry skin' since
early childhood,
as had his father
and brother.
a. What is the
   probable
   diagnosis?
b. How can the
   diagnosis be
   confirmed?

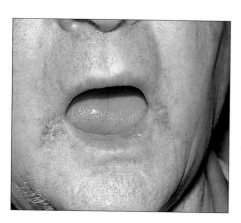

This patient has an
irritable eruption at
the angles of the
mouth.
a. What is the likely
   diagnosis?
b. What organism
   may be present?
c. What is the likely
   cause?

94 ▶

This woman complained of painful swellings on the sides of her feet when standing. No abnormality was present when lying flat but, on standing, these small nodules appeared.

a. What is the diagnosis?

b. Is a skin biopsy required?

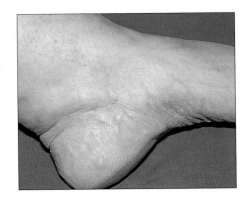

95 ▶

The lesion on this patient's forehead is of a few months' duration.

a. Describe the lesion.

b. What is the likely diagnosis?

c. What test is required?

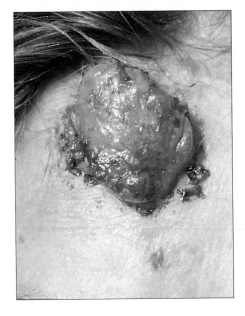

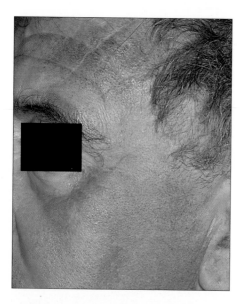

◀ 96
This man developed facial pigmentation.
a. What are the possible causes?

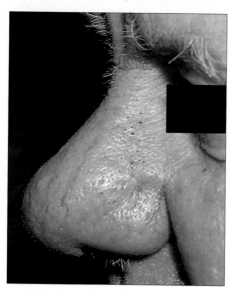

◀ 97
The nasal lesions shown here are the results of two different disorders.
a. What three abnormalities are illustrated?
b. What is the name of the disorder causing enlargement of the nose?
c. Which of the lesions shown are not a part of this diagnosis?

98 ▶

The patient in this illustration has an itchy rash.

a. What abnormality is shown?

b. How would you confirm the diagnosis?

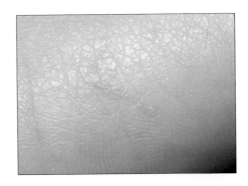

99 ▶

The illustration shows a hard papule on the heel of an infant.

a. Why is this lesion hard?

b. What is the cause?

c. What is the prognosis?

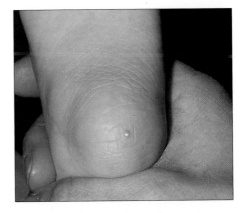

100 ▶

This woman's thumbnail kept splitting down the middle.

a. What is the probable diagnosis?

b. What is the prognosis?

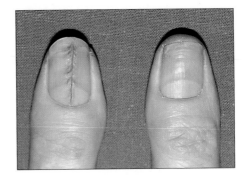

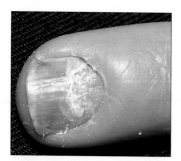

◀ **101**
This patient developed nail changes and swelling of the skin around several fingernails.
a. What features are shown?
b. What is the differential diagnosis?

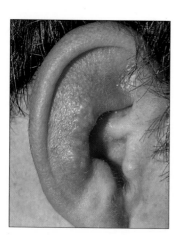

◀ **102**
The illustration shows an ear lesion in a young man.
a. What is the diagnosis?
b. How has this happened?

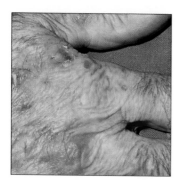

◀ **103**
These are blisters and skin fragility of recent onset on the exposed skin of a middle-aged man.
a. What is the likely diagnosis?
b. What causative factors should be considered?
c. What abnormal laboratory tests are likely?

104 ▶

This woman was concerned about the brown papules on her cheeks.
a. What is the cause?
b. What investigations are required?

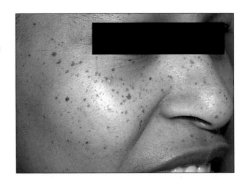

105 ▶

This child has suffered with a nodule on the lip for two months. The nodule bleeds frequently.
a. What is the likely diagnosis?
b. Where else may this lesion occur?
c. What is the treatment?

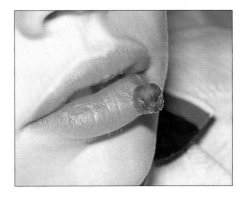

106 ▶

The patient shown here complains of a lesion on the eyelid.
a. What abnormality is shown?
b. Give three possible causes.

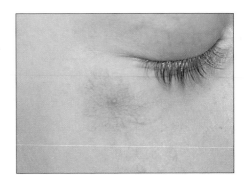

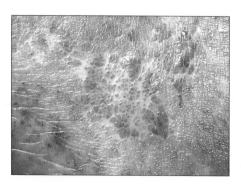

◄ 107

This patient complains of a painful area above the medial malleolus.

a. What is the name of this condition?

b. As part of what condition does it occur?

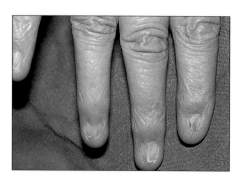

◄ 108

This woman and her daughter both presented with dystrophic nails and absent thumbnails.

a. What features are shown?

b. What is the most likely diagnosis?

c. What other features would you look for?

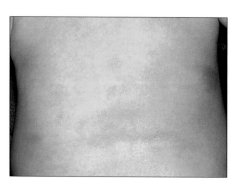

◄ 109

The mother of this child was concerned about the blue mark that appeared on its back.

a. What is the cause?

b. What investigations are required?

110 ►

This 60-year-old woman presents with asymptomatic changes of the left areola.

a. What is the likely diagnosis?

b. Name three other disorders which may cause erythema and crusting of the areola.

c. What clinical features are likely to distinguish them from this case?

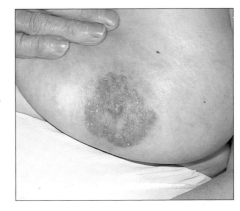

111 ►

The illustration shows an acute eruption on the neck of a farmer.

a. What is the likely diagnosis?

b. From which animal is it acquired?

c. How would you treat this?

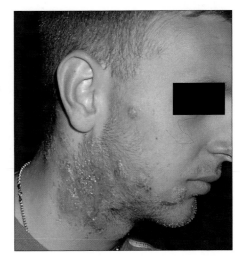

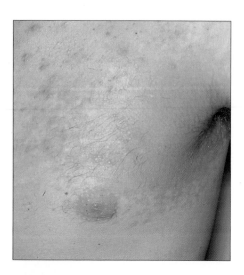

◄ **112**
This teenager complained of a brown, hairy area on the left side of his chest.
a. What is the diagnosis?
b. What is the prognosis?

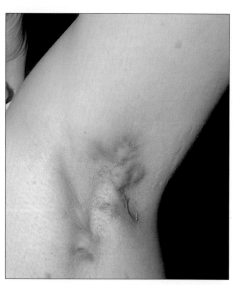

◄ **113**
This patient suffers from discharging lesions in the axillae and the perineal region.
a. What is the likely diagnosis?
b. If confined to the perineum, what other differential diagnoses should be considered?
c. With which other skin disorder may this be associated?

114 ▶

This tumour has been present for just two months.

a. What is the differential diagnosis?
b. How should it be managed?

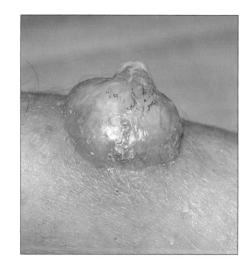

115 ▶

There is an area of discolouration on this patient's neck.

a. Describe the changes shown.
b. Of which chronic dermatosis is this a feature?
c. What name may be given to this manifestation?

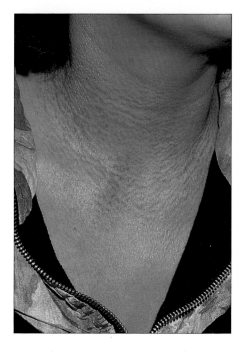

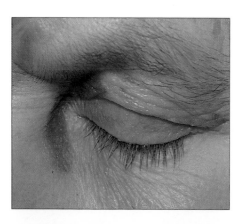

◄ 120

This patient had renal failure and cardiomegaly. She developed these purpuric areas around her eyes after rubbing them.

a. What is the diagnosis?

b. What other features should be looked for?

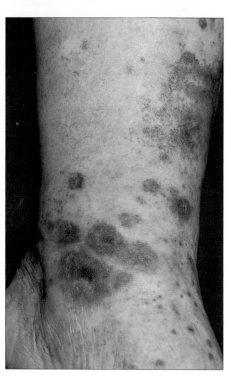

◄ 121

This man suffers from painful joints and blood in his urine.

a. What is the diagnosis?

b. What are the possible causes?

122 ▶

This dark band was found on the heel of a young man.

a. What is the name of this condition?

b. How is it caused?

c. With what may it be confused?

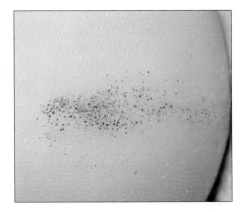

123 ▶

This child has been brought to the clinic suffering from itchy nodules on the arm.

a. These nodules are iatrogenic; what is the likely cause?

b. The chemical responsible is a metal. Which metal is it?

c. How would you avoid this problem?

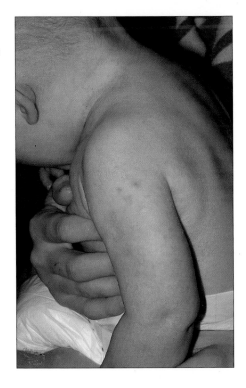

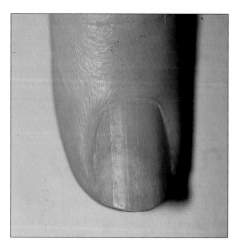

◀ **124**

An example of dystrophic nail is shown here.

a. What abnormalities can be seen?

b. Give four possible causes.

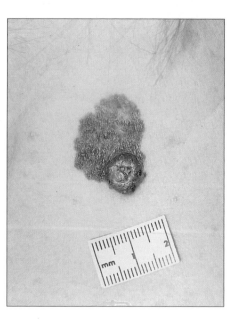

◀ **125**

The illustration shows a lesion on the neck of a patient.

a. Describe the appearances.

b. What is the likely diagnosis?

126 ▶

This child has had the mark on his scalp, seen here, since he was born.

a. What is the diagnosis?

b. What is the prognosis?

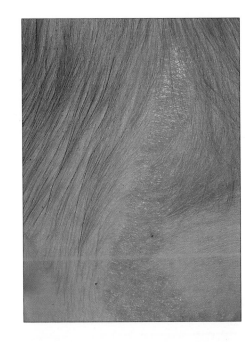

127 ▶

The lesion on this man's chest occurred a few days after a minor abrasion.

a. Describe the appearance.

b. What is the likely diagnosis?

c. What symptom would you expect to be present?

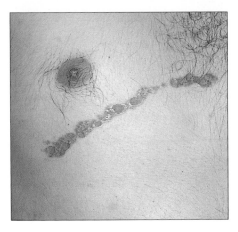

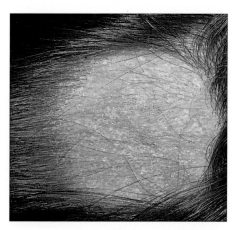

◄ 128

This boy developed a patch of hair loss.

a. What is the likely diagnosis, and why?

b. How would you make a definitive diagnosis?

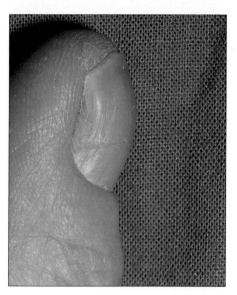

◄ 129

The illustration shows an abnormal nail in a man with a chronic medical disorder.

a. Describe the changes illustrated.

b. What is the name of this syndrome?

c. What is the likely associated disorder?

130 ▶

This child was brought to the clinic because of severe atopic eczema, seen on his cheek and around his ear. The skin tag in front of his ear was an incidental finding.

a. What is this lesion?

b. Does it have any significance?

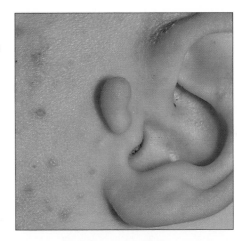

131 ▶

Three days after completing a course of ampicillin for a sore throat, this man developed a generalised rash.

a. Could this rash be due to the antibiotic?

b. What is the most relevant differential diagnosis?

c. Would you give him penicillin again?

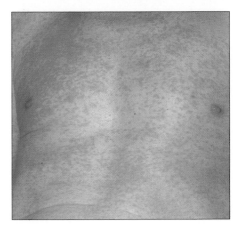

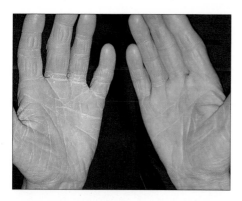

◄ 132
This man had a scaly rash on one hand.
a. What is the differential diagnosis?
b. What other body site should be examined?
c. What test would you do?

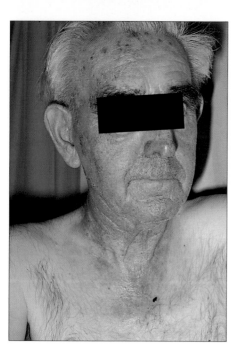

◄ 133
This male patient developed an acute rash on his face and the 'V' of his neck.
a. Name two possible groups of causes.
b. The rash was due to his systemic medication; name at least three likely culprits.

134 ▶

This woman, 38 weeks pregnant, complains of a crop of blisters.

a. What is the most likely diagnosis?

b. What are the risks to mother and foetus?

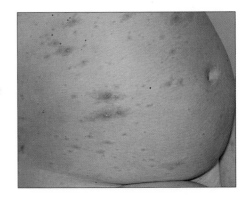

135 ▶

The illustration shows an acutely tender thumb in a child. The child also has a sore area on the lip.

a. What is the likely diagnosis for the two sites which are affected?

b. What is the name of the thumb condition?

c. What differential diagnosis should be considered?

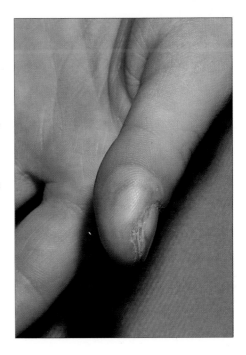

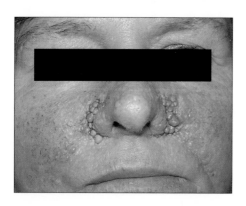

This woman's son suffered from epilepsy.
a. In the case of the woman, what is the diagnosis?
b. What other cutaneous features would you look for?

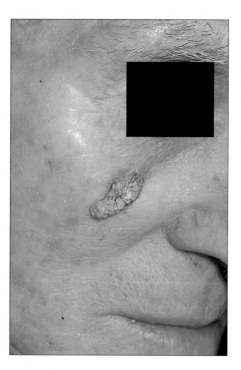

◄ 137
The illustration shows a lesion on the cheek of this elderly man.
a. How would you describe the lesion?
b. Name four possible diagnoses which may cause this clinical presentation.

138 ▶

This is a close-up view of the posterior nail fold of a man who presented with muscle weakness, and a rash on his face and hands.

a. What features are seen?

b. What is the probable diagnosis?

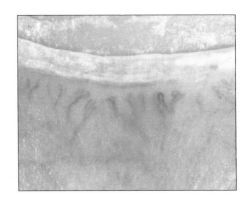

139 ▶

This patient has a number of melanocytic naevi on the legs.

a. What two important features are illustrated?

b. What is the name of this condition?

c. What is its importance?

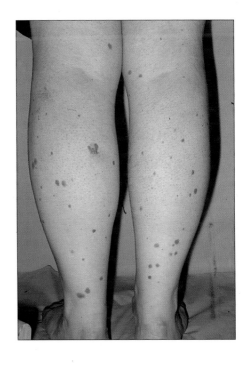

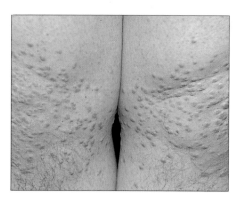

◀ 140

This man was referred with a rash on his knees. Close examination revealed multiple small yellow/orange papules on the knees, buttock and forearms.

a. What is the diagnosis?
b. What blood tests would confirm the diagnosis?

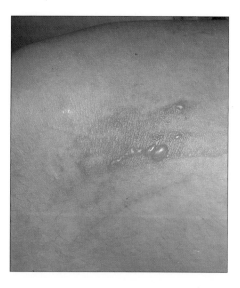

◀ 141

These itchy lesions were found on the skin of a child.

a. What important diagnostic feature is illustrated?
b. What is the likely diagnosis?
c. What residual effect may be visible when the inflammation settles?

142 ▶

This patient developed a rapidly swelling, tender leg.

a. What is the diagnosis?

b. How is this treated?

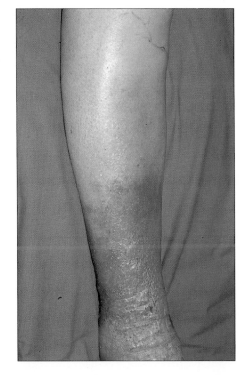

143 ▶

The teenage girl shown here has an acute skin eruption.

a. What is the diagnosis?

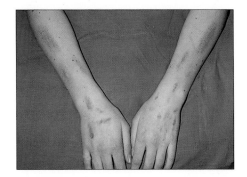

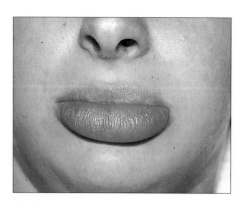

◀ **144**

This young child developed chronic lip swelling, which was worse on the lower lip.

a. Describe the features illustrated.

b. What possible causes must be considered?

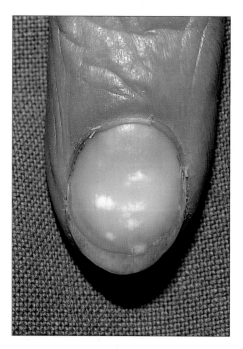

◀ **145**

The illustration demonstrates a common nail abnormality.

a. What is this appearance called?

b. What is its significance?

146 ▶

There is a striking abnormality to be found on this woman's trunk.

a. What is the diagnostically important physical sign illustrated?

b. What factors may enhance the effect of sun exposure?

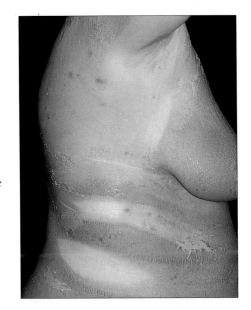

147 ▶

These lesions of a few months duration were found on the trunk of a child.

a. What is the likely diagnosis?

b. What useful diagnostic features are illustrated?

c. What is the prognosis?

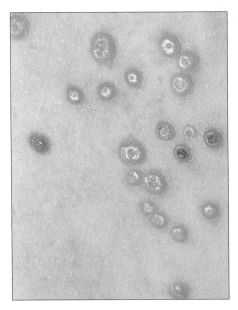

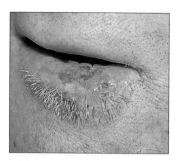

◄ 148

This elderly man presented with a hard nodule on his lower lip.

a. What is the diagnosis?

b. What is the risk of metastasis?

c. How could this be treated?

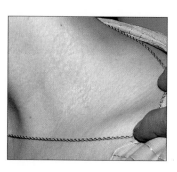

◄ 149

This patient reports a long-standing skin change of the neck and axilla.

a. Describe the physical signs.

b. What is the likely diagnosis?

c. What systemic features may occur?

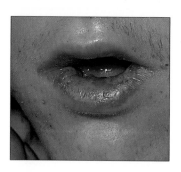

◄ 150

This young man has blistered lips and erosions of the penis, with acute onset; a similar episode occurred one year previously.

a. What is the likely diagnosis?

b. Name some likely causes of these eruptions.

c. Why is this unlikely to be herpetic gingivostomatitis?

151 ▶

The illustration shows lesions on the leg of an elderly woman.

a. What abnormality is shown?

b. What complications may occur?

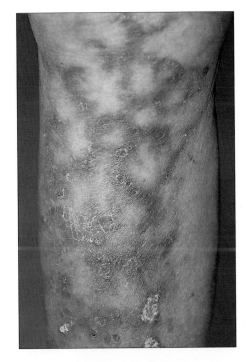

152 ▶

This patient developed a sore patch on the buccal mucosa.

a. What is the diagnosis?

b. How would you investigate this?

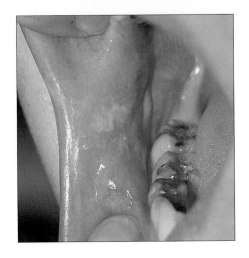

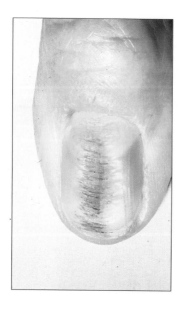

◀ **153**

The illustration shows an example of nail dystrophy dating back for a few years.

a. What is the cause of this abnormality?

b. What is the treatment?

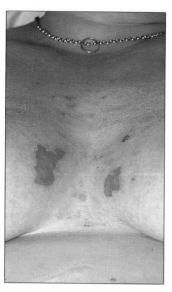

◀ **154**

This woman was being treated with penicillamine for rheumatoid arthritis. She developed patches on her skin which, she said, started as blisters.

a. Describe the lesions.

b. Is this caused by her penicillamine therapy?

155 ▶

This patient displays a congenital pigmented lesion.

a. What is the common name of this lesion?

b. What is its significance?

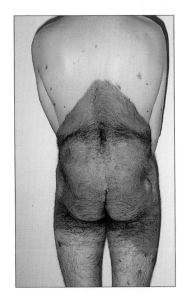

156 ▶

This primigravid patient, 39 weeks pregnant, has intensely itchy, urticated, erythematous papules, which start on her abdomen and spread to other sites.

a. What is the probable diagnosis?

b. Is there any risk to her unborn child?

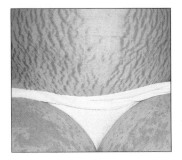

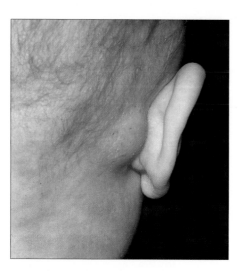

A retroauricular nodule is shown here, in an atopic child.

a. What is the likely nature of the nodule?
b. Why has it occurred?
c. How would you treat this?

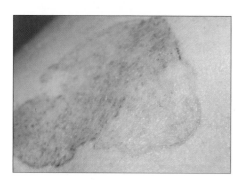

◀ 158

This man has had a slow-growing plaque, approximately 20 cm in diameter, on his trunk for several years.

a. What is the characteristic of the edge of the plaque?
b. What is the diagnosis?

159 ▶

A man complains of staining of his clothing in the axillary region.

a. What features are visible?

b. What is this disorder called, and what is the cause?

c. How would you treat it?

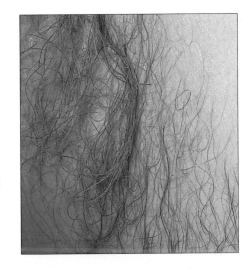

160 ▶

This patient had suffered from a widespread rash for years. Gradually the involved area became greater, individual plaques became thicker, and some started to ulcerate.

a. What is the diagnosis?

b. How can this be treated?

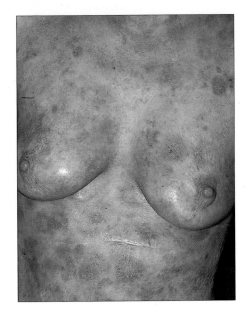

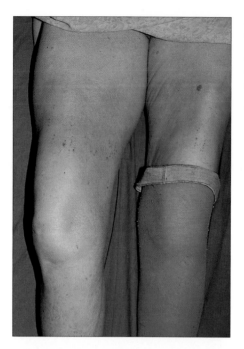

◀ **161**
This woman complains of an itchy rash on the thighs.
a. What is the likely cause?
b. What tests should be performed?

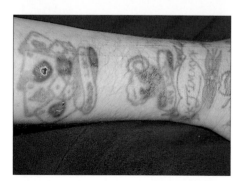

◀ **162**
This man developed itchy areas within the red parts of his tattoo.
a. What is the cause?
b. How is this treated?

163 ▶

The illustration shows abnormal scars on the knees of this patient after orthopaedic surgery.

a. What is the name of this type of scar?

b. What is the likely outcome of excising these scars?

c. What advice would you give to the patient about vaccinations?

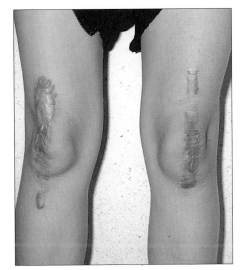

164 ▶

This child has suddenly developed crusted lesions on her face.

a. What is the diagnosis?

b. Should she go to school today?

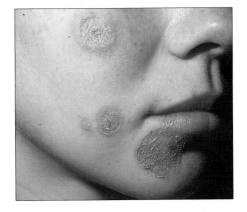

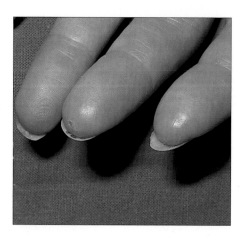

◀ **165**

This illustration shows fingertip lesions related to a systemic disorder.

a. What abnormality is shown?

b. What is the likely underlying disorder?

c. What other changes may occur in these digits?

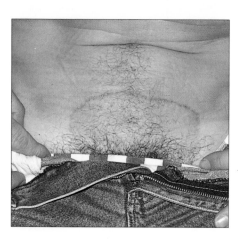

◀ **166**

This patient complains of a pubic rash of several months duration.

a. What is the likely diagnosis?

b. What other body site should be examined?

c. How might you identify the causative organism?

167 ▶

This patient suffers with photosensitivity, rash on the arms and erythema of the cheeks.

a. What is the likely diagnosis?

b. The patient had negative anti-nuclear antibody; what other test should be done?

c. What is the most frequent extra-cutaneous symptom?

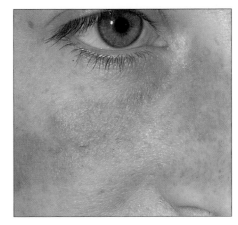

168 ▶

This man had a mole behind his knee for years. It has recently started to change colour.

a. What abnormal features are visible?

b. What is the probable diagnosis?

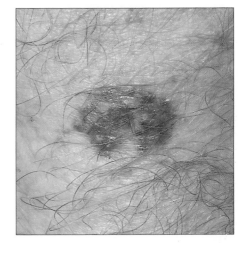

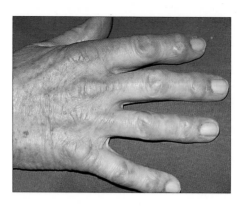

The illustration shows a rash on this patient's hands, and abnormal nail folds. The patient also has rash on the eyelids.
a. What is the likely diagnosis?
b. What musculo-skeletal symptom is likely?
c. What investigations should be performed?

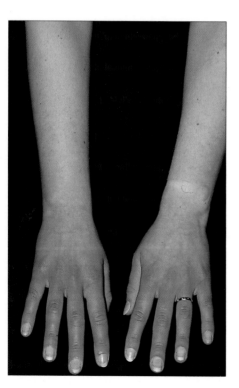

This young woman is concerned about the purple colour of her hands and feet.
a. What is the diagnosis?
b. What investigations would you perform?

171 ▶

This child has thickened encrustations on her scalp.

a. What feature is shown?

b. What is the differential diagnosis?

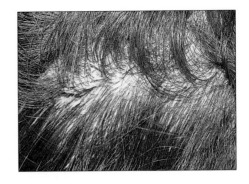

172 ▶

These eczematous lesions were found on the hand of a hospital in-patient.

a. What is the cause of this eruption?

b. What test may identify the causative chemical?

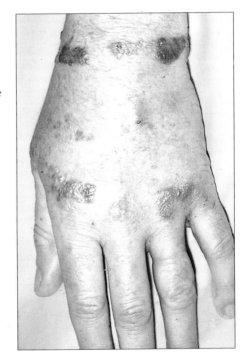

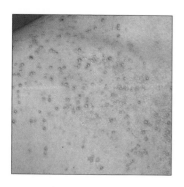

◀ 173

This young man, who was under the care of a general physician, suddenly developed multiple small, yellow pustules on his trunk and back.

a. What is the differential diagnosis?

b. This was not an infection and his lipids were normal. What is the probable cause?

c. How is this different from simple acne vulgaris?

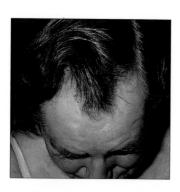

◀ 174

This is the scalp of a middle-aged woman with a three-month history of hirsutism.

a. What abnormality is shown?

b. What is the likely cause?

c. What initial investigations should be performed?

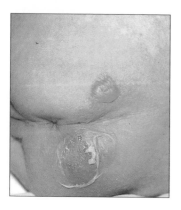

◀ 175

This two-day-old baby started to develop blisters on the backs of the fingers, buttocks and knees within hours of birth.

a. What is the probable diagnosis?

b. What is the prognosis?

c. What other diagnoses should be considered?

176 ►

This teenage boy presented with a history of asymptomatic marks on his back.

a. What are these marks and why have they occurred?
b. With what may they be confused?
c. What will happen to them?

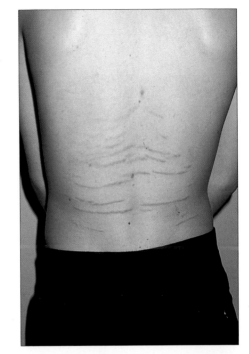

177 ►

This patient has symmetrical, largely asymptomatic, palmar eruptions.

a. What is the likely diagnosis?
b. What are the likely differential diagnoses?
c. What are the most important diagnostic features?

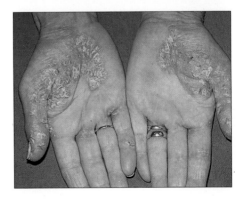

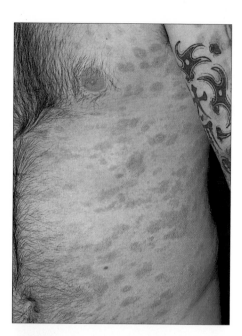

◀ **178**

This man presented with an itchy rash of sudden onset.

a. What is the probable diagnosis.

b. What question would you ask the patient to support your diagnosis?

c. What other diagnosis must always be considered?

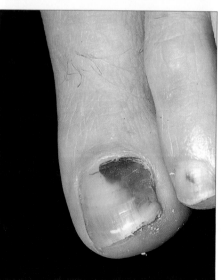

◀ **179**

The illustration shows a toenail lesion of two month's duration.

a. What is the likely diagnosis?

b. What reassuring features are present?

180 ▶

This woman suffers from a painful ulceration of the leg, of acute onset.

a. What is the likely diagnosis?

b. What types of associated systemic disease may be present?

c. Other than corticosteroids, which immunosuppressive drug is particularly helpful for treatment of this condition?

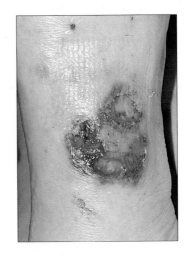

181 ▶

The female patient shown here has gradually developed widespread hair loss.

a. What examination features would you look for?

b. What are the causes of diffuse alopecia?

c. What investigations would you make?

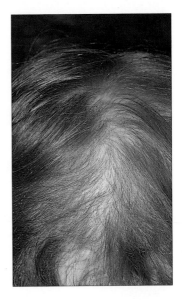

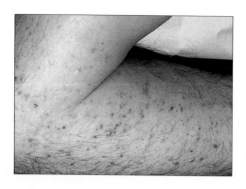

◄ 182

The illustration shows an incidental finding on the arm of a retired miner.

a. Describe the lesions shown.

b. What is their likely nature?

c. How have they been caused?

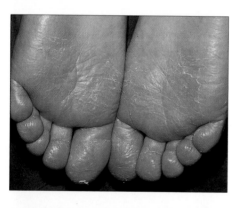

◄ 183

This child has persistent redness, splitting and cracking of the soles of the feet. The symptoms are worse at the ball of the foot.

a. What is the differential diagnosis?

b. What is the most likely diagnosis?

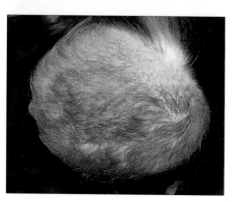

◄ 184

This young girl has developed extensive balding.

a. What abnormality is shown?

b. What is the differential diagnosis?

185 ▶

This female patient has extensive superficial blistering as a result of the administration of medication.

a. What is the name of this condition?

b. Which drugs may be implicated?

c. What ocular complication may ensue?

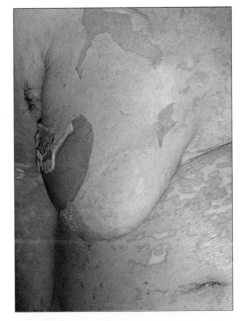

186 ▶

This woman complained of smelly feet, and had been treated for warts.

a. What feature is shown?

b. What is the cause of this condition?

c. How should it be treated?

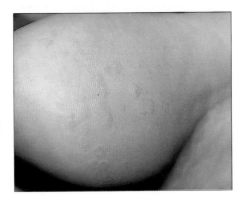

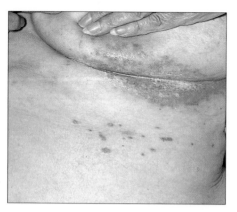

◀ 187
This in-patient, who also has a sore mouth, displays an inflammary rash.
a. What name describes this pattern of eruption?
b. What is the likely connection with the sore mouth?
c. What important diagnostic feature is illustrated?

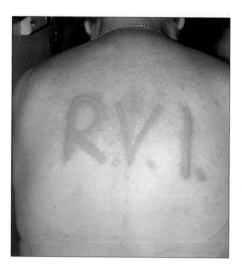

◀ 188
A classic example of writing on the skin is demonstrated in this picture.
a. What is the proper name for this condition?
b. To what group of disorders does it belong?
c. What is the underlying cause?

189 ▶

This patient has multiple scaly patches on her arms and legs. A diagnosis of actinic keratosis was considered, but rejected on closer examination.
a. What feature is shown?
b. What is the diagnosis?

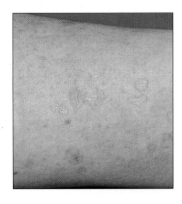

190 ▶

This woman has an asymptomatic lesion on the chin.
a. What is the likely diagnosis?
b. What investigations should be performed?

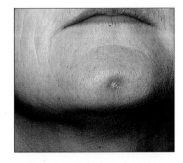

191 ▶

This man has developed nodules in a birth mark.
a. What is the diagnosis?
b. Why have the nodules appeared?
c. How could this be treated?

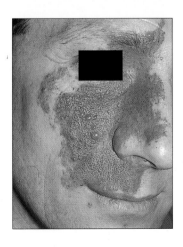

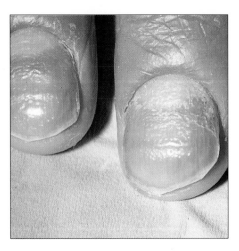

◀ **192**

The illustration shows the nails of a patient with long-standing skin disease.

a. What abnormalities are visible?

b. What is the likely cause?

c. What other disorders cause nail pitting?

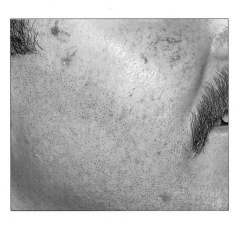

◀ **193**

This man complained of dilated blood vessels on his face.

a. What is the diagnosis?

b. What symptoms would you ask about?

c. What other features would you look for?

194 ▶

This is a solitary lesion of lengthy duration on the leg of an elderly woman.

a. What is the likely diagnosis?

b. Some patients have multiple lesions; with which common dermatosis may they be confused?

c. What is the likely cause in a patient with multiple lesions and with keratoses on the palms of the hands?

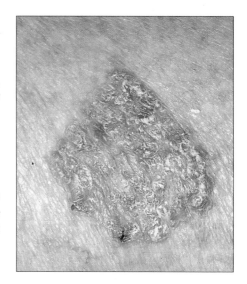

195 ▶

This woman demonstrates a drug-induced hypertrichosis.

a. Name at least three drugs which may cause this disorder.

b. In a female with no relevant drug history, what physical signs would alert you to the possibility of an androgen-secreting tumour?

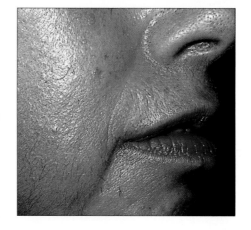

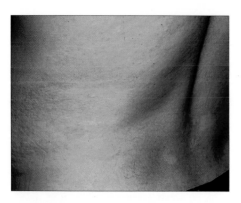

◀ **196**
This mentally deficient patient has these changes on the trunk.
a. What is the diagnosis?
b. How would you demonstrate one feature more clearly?

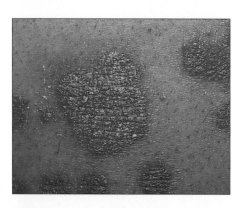

◀ **197**
Widespread red scaly patches are found on the trunk and limbs of this man.
a. What is the most likely diagnosis?
b. What topical treatments are available?

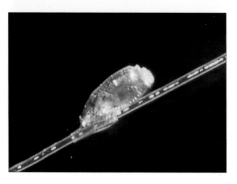

◀ **198**
This is a hair taken from a child with an itchy scalp.
a. What feature is shown?
b. How is this treated?

199 ▶

This man had
treated the eczema
on his face for years
using a cream.
a. What has
   happened?
b. Can anything be
   done about it?

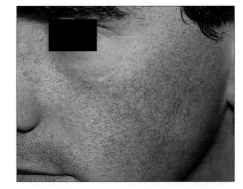

200 ▶

This patient suffers
from a chronic
eruption on the
soles of the feet.
a. What is the likely
   diagnosis?
b. What differential
   diagnosis is im-
   portant if this is
   asymmetrical?
c. In what ways
   might the social
   history be of
   importance?

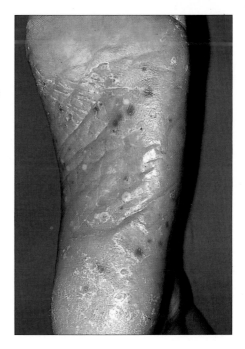

ANSWERS

1 a. There are multiple crusted and eroded areas on his head, neck and upper trunk.

 b. Acute eczema; impetigo; pemphigus foliaceous. The crusty and oozy lesions are characteristic of subacute eczema, where exudate leaks through the skin. Although secondary infection is common, the example shown in this illustration is unlikely to be one of staphylococcal impetigo because the exudate is more viscous and lesions less oedematous. The intra-epidermal blisters of pemphigus foliaceous and erythematosus are so fragile that they burst easily, leaving only crusted and eroded lesions.

2 a. Reiter's syndrome; the manifestation illustrated is keratoderma blenorrhagica.

 b. Urethra or gastrointestinal tract.

 c. Arthritis, conjunctivitis, balanitis, oral lesions, rarely cardiac or neurological manifestations.

3 a. These are angiomas in the skin. Blue-rubber bleb naevus and congenital multiple glomus tumours both cause this type of lesion and both conditions are inherited as an autosomal dominant. The difference can be established by skin biopsy. The two conditions must be distinguished because blue-rubber bleb syndrome is associated with systemic, potentially fatal, angiomas, whereas multiple glomus tumours are not.

 b. If thrombosis occurs, the resulting black and brown colours may be confused with melanocyte-derived tumours.

4 a. Geographic tongue, or migratory glossitis.

 b. None, apart from symptoms (pain or burning); most cases are idiopathic.

 c. Pustular psoriasis; Reiter's syndrome.

5 a. Epidermoid cyst.

 b. Epidermoid cysts are lined by keratinizing epithelium. The degenerating keratinous contents produce the foul smell. These cysts are not derived from sebaceous glands but are frequently incorrectly called sebaceous cysts.

6 a. Lichen sclerosus et atrophicus (also termed balanitis xerotica obliterans when the penis is affected).

b. Reduced support of blood vessels due to changes in upper dermal collagen.

c. Often none; there may be burning, irritation, tightness, phimosis, paraphimosis, or altered urinary stream if the meatus is involved.

7 a. Post-scabetic nodules. These occur in approximately 4% of infected individuals, and may last for six months after the infection has been adequately treated.

b. No. The nodules are believed to be due to an inflammatory reaction to retained mite antigens, but they are not a sign of persistent infection.

8 a. Lichen planus.

b. Koebner's phenomenon (lesions localising to a minor injury); Wickham's striae (white marks within the lesions).

c. Examine the mouth; mucosal lesions are present in 75% of patients.

9 a. Erysipelas or cellulitis of the face. This is distinguished from acute facial eczema by the associated systemic features of fever, high erythrocyte sedimentation rate (ESR) and, in retrospect, a raised antistreptolysin O (ASOT) titre.

b. Culture of skin swabs, aspiration of tissue fluid or skin biopsy specimens rarely result in culture of the causative organism – *Streptococcus pyogenes* Lancefield Group A.

10 a. Oral hairy leukoplakia; lichen planus.

b. AIDS; this appearance, together with nodules on the legs, could be due to lichen planus, but similar palatal nodules make AIDS with Kaposi's sarcoma the more likely diagnosis.

11 a. Insect-bite reactions (papular urticaria). There are multiple grouped papules which show pronounced post-inflammatory pigmentation in this case.

b. Grouped insect bites on relatively non-exposed sites are usually due to fleas (animal or human) or body lice. Bites appearing principally on exposed sites are generally due to flying insects (e.g. mosquitoes).

12 a. Atrophic scars with secondary purpura.

b. Ehlers–Danlos syndrome.

c. Hypermobile joints.

13 a. As well as the black streak, which runs the entire length of the nail plate, there is pigment on the posterior nail fold (Hutchinson's sign).

   b. Nail pigment streaks are common in Afro-Caribbeans, but are abnormal in whites. The combination of a solitary pigmented nail streak and pigmentation of the posterior nail fold is diagnostic of a melanoma affecting the nail matrix, with migration of pigment cells on to the posterior nail fold.

   c. Longitudinal nail biopsy through the streak will confirm the diagnosis.

14 a. Discrete, inflammatory, crusted, coin-sized plaques.

   b. Discoid (nummular) eczema. Inflammatory psoriasis is a possibility, but the lesions are usually more annular and slower in evolution; secondary infection of an underlying itchy rash such as scabies should be considered, but the lesions shown are rather too discrete for this to be a strong possibility.

   c. Administration of a potent topical corticosteroid; treatment of any secondary infection.

15 a. There is unilateral redness and scaling of the skin on her right foot, with a well-defined scaly edge best seen on the lower leg.

   b. Tinea incognito. When a skin fungal infection is inadvertently treated with potent topical steroids the rash appears to improve initially as the topical steroid inhibits the normal inflammatory response to the fungus.

16 a. Parasitophobia; debris of various types is presented under Sellotape or in a matchbox.

   b. Microscopy, to ensure that there are no parasites visible.

   c. Pimozide.

17 a. There is rather diffuse thickening of the skin overlying the dorsum of the proximal phalanx, with typical peau d'orange appearance.

   b. Pretibial myxoedema.

   c. Thyroid acropachy. This, in conjunction with pretibial myxoedema and exophthalmus, constitutes Diamond's triad.

18 a. Vitiligo; industrial leucoderma may be considered, but is much less common and is unlikely to have foci of repigmentation, as illustrated here.

   b. Other organ-specific auto-immune disorders may be present (or their corresponding antibody tests may be positive), but screening for these in apparently healthy individuals is of debatable relevance.

   c. Both; to the white areas to prevent burning, and to the normal (brown) skin to decrease the accentuation between this and the affected skin by stopping it tanning.

19 a. Superficial spreading malignant melanoma.

   b. Excision of the suspect mole with a 2mm margin of normal skin through fat is indicated in the first instance. Histological examination of the entire specimen will enable confirmation of the diagnosis and measurement of the tumour depth. At present it is suggested that tumours less than 2mm thick should be excised down to deep fascia with a 10mm margin, and thicker tumours with a 30mm margin. Further study will inevitably affect these recommendations.

20 a. Scaly brown lesion with a serpiginous pattern.

   b. Cutaneous larva migrans.

   c. Larva of the canine hookworm, due to contact with dog faeces, probably encountered on the beach.

21 a. Broken livedo. There are patches of purpuric mottling which correspond to the normal skin vascular pattern. This mottling is fixed and does not blanch. The distribution is quite different from the uniform physiological mottling (see case 71), and is always pathological.

   b. The combination of central nervous system symptoms and broken livedo suggests either arteriosclerosis, polyarteritis nodosa, systemic lupus erythematosus or emboli caused by thrombocythaemia or cholesterol crystals.

22 a. Seborrhoeic eczema.

   b. 'Cradle cap'.

   c. The prognosis is good; the eruption upsets the parents rather than the child and will resolve. If itch is prominent, this may indicate that the child has atopic eczema, which is more persistent.

23 a. There are several target-shaped lesions on the palm.

   b. These are characteristic – but not diagnostic – of erythema multiforme. Target lesions are also seen in urticaria, vasculitis and lupus erythematosus.

   c. Causes of erythema multiforme include: infections (viral: Herpes simplex, mycoplasma; bacterial: focal sepsis; fungal: coccidiomycosis); drugs (sulphonamides, anticonvulsants); and systemic disease (pregnancy, malignancy, radiotherapy). In many cases no cause is found.

24 a. Basal-cell carcinoma; granuloma fissuratum (possibly due to the rubbing of spectacles). The latter was the diagnosis in this case.
   b. The patient should be asked if he regularly wears spectacles.
   c. An incisional biopsy may be required to exclude malignancy.

25 a. Possible diagnoses include: pustular psoriasis; necrolytic migratory erythema; candida; pustular exanthem; drug eruption; bullous disease, e.g. pemphigus foliaceous.
   b. This was pustular psoriasis – the combination of systemic symptoms and lesions with peripheral pustules is characteristic. Oral retinoids (acitretin) or methotrexate are the drugs of choice in patients whose rash does not resolve spontaneously.

26 a. Twisted hairs, perifollicular purpura.
   b. This is likely to be ascorbic acid deficiency (scurvy). In this case, it was a consequence of living alone and having a poor diet.

27 a. Scalp psoriasis. Hyperkeratotic scaling, sharply demarcated from the adjacent, unaffected scalp, is characteristic of psoriasis and unlike seborrhoeic eczema of the scalp, in which the entire scalp is diffusely affected.
   b. Look for well-defined plaques with a predilection for the extensor surfaces, nail changes (pitting, onycholysis, and thickening), and flexural involvement.

28 a. Tinea pedis ('athlete's foot').
   b. Microscopy and culture of skin scrapings.

29 a. Urticaria.
   b. Urticaria may be due to allergic reactions (drugs and foodstuffs), auto-immune disease (systemic lupus erythematosus), physical stimuli (cholinergic urticaria, cold urticaria, etc.) or parasitic infections. In most cases no cause can be found. In the absence of other symptoms or signs, or a history suggestive of a physical urticaria or possible allergic cause, further investigation is likely to prove fruitless.

30 a. Purpuric spots on the pre-septal skin of the eyelid.
   b. Severe coughing or retching (in this case the precipitating factor was coughing episodes over two days).

31 a. There is a red, scaling plaque with prominent follicular plugging and scarring.

b. These are all features of discoid lupus erythematosus, which also produces patchy, scarring alopecia.

32 a. Herpes zoster (shingles).
b. Urinary retention, due to pain on attempted micturition.
c. Post-herpetic neuralgia, ulceration, secondary infection, motor nerve involvement in the leg (rarely).

33 a. Exfoliative dermatitis.
b. Possible causes include: drug eruption (gold, isoniazid); psoriasis; eczema (contact, atopic, seborrhoeic); reticulosis (leukaemia, Sézary syndrome); rarities (pityriasis rubra pilaris, ichthyiosiform erythroderma, pemphigus erythematosus, lichen planus, scabies).
c. Potential immediate complications result from: increased skin blood flow (heat loss and risk of hypothermia); high-output cardiac failure; increased cell turnover (protein loss through exfoliation); reduced barrier function due to abnormal stratum corneum (increased percutaneous water loss leading to dehydration); and associated gut changes (mild malabsorption).

34 a. Atopic dermatitis.
b. Family history of atopic disorders (a personal history of other atopic disorders would not normally be found in the age group illustrated); typical distribution and morphology of lesions; variation over a period of time; itch.
c. Herpes simplex, causing eczema herpeticum.

35 a. There are multiple short 'exclamation mark' hairs with narrow depigmented base and broader, pigmented, broken end.
b. Alopecia areata.
c. Other features of alopecia areata include: black dots or cadaverized hairs (these occur when the hair follicle is so badly damaged by the inflammatory process that only the products of follicle degeneration remain); patchy hair loss at other body sites; fine pitting on the finger nails.

36 a. Seborrhoeic warts or keratoses; basal-cell papillomas.
b. No. There is a paraneoplastic form (the sign of Leser–Trelat), but in such cases the lesions are itchy, eruptive and small rather than the larger, long-standing lesions illustrated here.

37 a. Symmetrical scaling, crusting and redness of the skin around the lip, a sharp demarcation from the adjacent skin and normal vermilion.

b. These changes are characteristic of a lip-licking dermatitis in which salivary enzymes produce maceration and irritant eczema of the perioral tissues, without damaging the saliva-resistant lips. Contact allergic reactions to foodstuffs and toothpastes usually produce changes most marked at the corners of the mouth. Lipstick or lip salve allergy will produce similar changes, but without the sharp demarcation from the uninvolved skin.

38 a. Unilocular, tense blisters, with serous or haemorrhagic fluid content, arising on a background of apparently normal skin.
   b. Bullous pemphigoid. Elderly age group, preceding itchy plaques, and the above morphology, are typical; mouth involvement is typical of pemphigus, but is only apparent in about 5% of patients with bullous pemphigoid.
   c. Skin biopsy for histology, including frozen sections for direct immunofluorescence tests.

39 a. Plane warts.
   b. Spontaneous resolution.
   c. Treatment is preferably by reassurance alone; sometimes mild peeling agents may be used.

40 a. These are neuropathic skin changes. The ulcer is on a weight-bearing portion of the foot, and has a hyperkeratotic, well-defined, edge.
   b. Blisters on the tips of the toes, or on callosities, are common initial features of diabetic neuropathy complicated by reduced blood flow, such as has occurred here. Neuropathic changes are seen in peripheral neuropathy (diabetes mellitus, leprosy) or spinal cord disease (poliomyelitis, syringomyelia, tabes dorsalis).

41 a. Strawberry naevus (capillary cavernous haemangioma).
   b. These are commonly present at birth or appear in the first few weeks of life. Thereafter, they slowly involute spontaneously, with 90% having gone by the age of nine years.
   c. Indications for treatment are when a large, periocular, strawberry naevus is obscuring vision, making feeding difficult, or causing significant platelet consumption due to intravascular coagulation within the haemangioma (Kasabach–Merritt syndrome).

42 a. Gangrene of the hallux.
   b. Diabetes mellitus.

43 a. There is hair loss in a band along the front of the scalp.

b. This is characteristic of a tractional alopecia. In this case, it was due to regular use of tight hairdressing rollers. Traction alopecia on the temple is seen in people who wear a long plait, or who wear their hair rolled up tight on the top of the head.

c. The changes are irreversible.

44 a. Xanthomatous deposits; gouty tophi; granuloma annulare (the most likely of the three in current dermatological practice).

b. Arthritis, swollen joints, or tophi elsewhere would be expected in cases of gouty tophi, which was the diagnosis in this case.

45 a. There are two areas of scarring alopecia in which the scalp skin is smooth, shiny and depressed, with no follicular orifices.

b. Aplasia cutis – a congenital absence of scalp skin resulting in ulceration at birth. Aplasia cutis may be an isolated finding, or may be associated with other congenital abnormalities.

46 a. This is liquid nitrogen cryotherapy, performed to treat warts.

b. It is painful, even if a relatively gentle application is performed.

47 a. Erythema nodosum.

b. Common causes include: bacterial infection (streptococci, tuberculosis); viral infection (mycoplasma, chlamydia, rickettsia); fungal infection (coccidiomycosis); drugs (sulphonamides, oral contraceptives); systemic disease (sarcoidosis, Crohn's disease and ulcerative colitis).

48 a. Xanthelasma.

b. Hyperlipidaemia (usually, hypercholesterolaemia).

c. Coronary artery disease.

49 a. Black hairy tongue.

b. The filiform papillae on the tongue become longer, for obscure reasons. Pigmentation is produced by bacteria coating the papillae. Precipitating factors include antibiotic therapy and administration of any drug that reduces saliva secretion, such as tricyclic antidepressants.

50 a. Dermatofibroma (pigmented histiocytoma).

b. The cause is unknown; insect bites have been suggested as a possible cause.

c. None; treatment is not required for asymptomatic lesions.

51 a. Carbuncle. *Staphylococcus aureus* infection of a group of adjacent hair follicles produces a painful, hard, red lump which suppurates after a period of five to seven days. Central skin necrosis occurs and a scar is often left.

  b. Predisposing factors include diabetes, malnutrition, steroid therapy and generalized dermatoses.

52 a. White skin, fusion of the labia.

  b. Dyspareunia, altered urinary flow.

  c. Lichen sclerosus et atrophicus.

53 a. Patch tests.

  b. This is a test for delayed lymphocyte-mediated hypersensitivity, i.e. contact allergic eczema. It is of no use for the investigation of most urticarial reactions or systemic drug reactions. Patch test materials are applied to the skin for 48 hours and the results read 48–96 hours later. A raised red patch or vesiculation indicates allergy to that allergen. In this case there are positive reactions to several constituents of rubber.

  c. They identify the position of individual allergens when the test strips are removed.

54 a. This is likely to be lichen planus.

  b. About 75%.

  c. Usually none, but may cause soreness or burning pain (but not itch).

55 a. Facial flushing is usually physiological (blushing), provoked by emotional stimuli. This usually involves the face, neck and chest, producing a transient, mottled redness. Other causes of facial flushing include alcohol (alone or in combination with chlor-propamide), disulfiram, solvent exposure (e.g. trichloroethylene, dimethylformamide), menopausal and endocrine/metabolic effects (adrenalin secreting phaeochromocytoma, carcinoid syndrome, mastocytosis).

56 a. Meningococcal meningitis.

  b. Members of the patient's immediate family should be given prophylactic rifampicin therapy.

57 a. There is purpura with incipient ulceration of the skin on his ears, cheeks and nose. These are peripheral facial sites where the effects of cooling are greatest.

b. This man had a cryoglobulinaemia. Cryo-precipitation had occurred, leading to widespread vasculitis and subsequent skin necrosis.

58 a. Acne excoriee, caused by picking at minor blemishes.
   b. In this age group, a significant proportion of patients suffer from depression.
   c. The lesions will leave permanent scars.

59 a. There are ivory white, wrinkly plaques of skin with well-developed follicular keratoses.
   b. This is probably lichen sclerosis et atrophicus.
   c. Similar changes with scarring (see case 52) are commonly present on the vulva and perianal skin.

60 a. The new rash is likely to be the result of contact allergy to an ear-drop.
   b. Antibiotics (especially neomycin), corticosteroids, preservatives.
   c. Patch testing.

61 a. There is a nodule with a depressed centre and a pearly edge, with telangiectasia.
   b. Nodular basal-cell carcinoma.
   c. Cryotherapy, radiotherapy, curettage and excision.

62 a. This is on the lateral aspect of the helix (rim) of the ear, at the upper pole; most actinic keratoses and squamous-cell carcinomas of the helix arise from the more fleshy superior or posterior parts of the helix rather than from the lateral border, as illustrated here.
   b. Chondrodermatitis nodularis helicis.

63 a. Mycetoma (Madura Foot).
   b. This is a deep fungal or actinomycetes infection of the soft tissues and bones, which may occur at any site but is most common on the foot and hand, where penetrating injuries introduce the organism. There are some 11 fungal and six actinomycetes species which can produce this clinical picture.

64 a. This is Giant Hogweed (*Heracleum mantegazzianum*). Related hedgerow species which cause a similar reaction include other hogweeds, cow parsley and chervil.
   b. Mainly along riverbanks in Scotland.
   c. The photosensitizing chemical is a psoralen, similar to that used in PUVA photochemotherapy.

65 a. There is blanching of the red skin around the scratch lines. This is called white dermographism, caused by vasoconstriction occurring after gentle scratching.
  b. It is typically seen in atopic patients, but also occurs in the inflamed skin of patients with psoriasis and other types of eczema.

66 a. There are multiple, small, keratotic lesions on a background of tanned atrophic skin.
  b. Solar (actinic) keratoses.
  c. On exposed sites, such as the face, forearms or scalp (if bald).

67 a. Condylomata acuminata.
  b. These are caused by human papilloma virus, probably acquired from the mother during a vaginal delivery. Sexual abuse must also be considered, and examination, under general anaesthetic if necessary, performed for evidence of rectal or vulval penetration and to take bacterial swabs for co-existing, potentially sexually transmitted organisms, e.g. gonococci, Chlamydia trachomatis, streptococci and staphylococci. HPV viral typing will demonstrate the viral type but not the way in which the infection was acquired.

68 a. Colonisation by *Pseudomonas*.
  b. This is unlikely; subungual colonization by this organism is usually a secondary phenomenon.

69 a. There are two plaques of atrophic, translucent, brownish skin on the anterior shins. Telangiectatic vessels and large veins are easily seen through the thin, atrophic skin.
  b. Necrobiosis lipoidica.
  c. Approximately 40% of patient with necrobiosis lipoidica do not have diabetes mellitus, although a high proportion have an abnormal glucose tolerance test. Only 0.3% of diabetics develop necrobiosis lipoidica. The presence of necrobiosis lipoidica is not related to the severity or control of the diabetes.

70 a. Acute paronychia.
  b. Usually *Staphylococcus aureus*; occasionally *Candida albicans* or Herpes simplex virus infection of the adjacent skin (herpetic whitlow).

71 a. Physiological vascular mottling. This is a normal appearance in the skin of younger people, especially in cold weather. It is commonly seen in small babies, and simply reflects the normal pattern of blood flow in the skin.

b. No investigation is required for this isolated finding. Compare this to the presentation and findings in case 21.

72 a. Granuloma annulare.
b. Ringworm lesions would be unlikely to be present at this size for a period of six months, and would have a scaling component.
c. The historical association with diabetes mellitus is very unusual for the common variants of this condition, but simple urinalysis for glucose in adults is reasonable as a safeguard.

73 a. Carcinoma of the vulva.
b. Lichen sclerosis et atrophicus (see case 52) produces itchy, white, atrophic plaques on the skin of the vulva, and results in atrophy of the labia majora, meatal stenosis and narrowing of the introitus – as in this patient. It has been estimated that approximately 5% of women with this condition will go on to develop squamous-cell carcinoma in the affected skin.

74 a. Fixed drug eruption.
b. Episodic inflammation, with eventual fixed pigmentation (due to melanin in dermal macrophages, rather than a primary melanocyte abnormality).
c. Sulphonamides, tetracyclines, barbiturates, salicylates, phenolphthalein.

75 a. Neurofibromatosis (von Recklinghausen's disease).
b. Autosomal dominant, but high frequency of sporadic mutation.
c. Kyphoscoliosis, bone cysts, fractures, bone hypertrophy, orbital defects.

76 a. Acne cysts, comedones and pustules.
b. Severe, scarring acne such as this is best treated with oral isotretinoin. Large cysts can be injected with triamcinolone in an attempt to reduce scarring.

77 a. Raynaud's phenomenon.
b. Idiopathic, collagen–vascular disorders (especially systemic sclerosis), arterial obstruction (external compression; vessel wall abnormalities such as arteriosclerosis or vasculitis; luminal occlusion by thrombi or due to blood hyperviscosity), neurological abnormalities affecting the limb, drugs (e.g. beta-blockers, nicotine, vinyl chloride, ergot).
c. Vibration White Finger.

78 a. Darier's disease – an autosomal-dominant condition.

b. Crusted papules, often confluent, variably involving the trunk, ears, and limbs, 'cobblestone' papules on the dorsum of the hands (acrodermatitis verucciformis), palmar pitting and nail changes.

79 a. This is likely to be threadworm infestation.
   b. Administer antihelminthic drug (e.g. mebendazole, thiabendazole, piperazine, pyrantel).
   c. Secondary bacterial infection; at this site in a child, suspect a Group A or Group G streptococcal infection.

80 a. Causes of the dystrophy seen here could include: dermatophyte infection of the nail plate; candida infection of the nail plate; ischaemic dystrophy of the elderly; psoriasis/eczema.
   b. Dermatophyte infection (Tinea unguium).
   c. Take clippings for microscopy and fungal culture.
   d. Systemic antifungal therapy. Topical treatment will not be adequate for this degree of involvement.

81 a. Pilar cysts are skin-coloured or rather paler, and overlying alopecia is not a feature (compare with case 5).
   b. Carcinoma of the bronchus, with scalp metastases.
   c. Urgent biopsy of scalp nodule, and chest radiogram.

82 a. Kaposi's sarcoma.
   b. This was classical Kaposi's sarcoma, in which the tumours are characteristically slow-growing, multiple purple macules as an isolated finding on the extremities of elderly men of African or Jewish origin. Patients from this group typically are not HIV-positive, and have no signs of immune suppression. Metastasis can occur to lymph nodes, and there may be marked lymphoedema in advanced cases.

83 a. Urticaria pigmentosa, a type of cutaneous mastocytosis.
   b. Release of histamine and other inflammatory mediators from mast cells give rise to the redness. This is Darier's sign.
   c. Slow spontaneous resolution is usual during childhood.

84 a. White streaks; distal nail splitting.
   b. This is Darier's disease, an autosomal-dominant disorder. Crusted, often confluent, keratotic papules may be present on the trunk, ears, and limbs. Cobblestone-shaped, confluent papules are found on the dorsum of the hands (acrodermatitis verucciformis).
   c. Palmar pitting is prominent.

85 a. Alopecia areata; selective sparing of white hairs is a common feature.
   b. No; skin pigmentation is not affected in this disorder. Vitiligo can cause patches of white hair and white skin but does not cause hair loss.

86 a. These are normal hypertrophic sebaceous glands in a healthy newborn child. Under the influence of maternal hormone stimulation, the child's sebaceous glands hypertrophy and produce increased quantities of sebum. The effect lasts for approximately six weeks; the sebaceous glands then regress, not appearing again until puberty. They should not be confused with obstructed immature sweat ducts producing miliaria in babies.

87 a. This is likely to be pityriasis versicolor.
   b. Take skin scrapings for microscopy, to visualize the causative yeast.
   c. The pigmentary disturbance may persist for several months, despite adequate treatment.

88 a. There are multiple pustules on the sole of the child's foot, with associated scale, papules and possible burrows, although the latter are not easily seen in this view.
   b. Scabies infections in babies commonly produce pustules on the soles of the feet.
   c. Identification of the adult mite or eggs will confirm the diagnosis; this is easier to obtain from an infested older sibling or parent.

89 a. Marked finger clubbing and cyanosis.
   b. Congenital cyanotic cardiovascular disease is the most likely cause of this combination in this age group. The patient had a haemoglobin concentration of 25g/dl.
   c. Respiratory (neoplasm; bronchiectasis/chronic infection); cardiac (endocarditis; atrial myxoma); gastrointestinal (cirrhosis; ulcerative colitis; Crohn's disease; coeliac disease); endocrine (thyrotoxicosis).

90 a. Congenital mal-alignment of the great toes; trauma; fungal infection.
   b. In childhood, dystrophic nails are usually due to a congenital malalignment of the nail, resulting in crooked nail growth into the lateral nail wall and, ultimately, ingrown toenail. Fungal infections produce a thickened but crumbly nail plate.

91 a. (Sutton's) halo naevus.
   b. The lesions are usually seen on the trunk, and are often multiple.

c. The de-pigmented area is at risk of sunburn, as it is unlikely to re-pigment within the timescale of a holiday.

92 a. Sex-linked recessive ichthyosis. There are large, dark, ichthyotic scales. The whole body is affected so that, unlike the autosomal-dominant ichthyosis vulgaris, some degree of flexural involvement is usually present.

b. Reduced aryl sulphate E and steroid sulphatase activity can be demonstrated in epidermis, fibroblast and leucocytes, and may be useful in diagnosis.

93 a. Angular stomatitis (angular cheilitis, perleche).

b. *Candida albicans.*

c. Usually loss of facial height due to age and/or worn-down dentures; deficiency of iron or vitamins is a much less common cause.

94 a. Painful piezogenic papules. These are a normal, sometimes painful, variant in which fat herniates through the dermis.

b. No further investigation is required; biopsy would just show normal skin.

95 a. Large, fleshy, crusted nodule.

b. Squamous-cell carcinoma (SCC); the short history is consistent with keratoacanthoma, but the morphology and lack of keratinisation suggest that this is a poorly differentiated SCC.

c. Diagnostic biopsy.

96 a. This fine, speckled, grey pigmentation is characteristic of minocycline-induced colour change. Similar appearances may occur with other drugs (amiodarone, gold, phenothiazines) and metals (argyria, mercury).

97 a. Enlarged nose (rhinophyma); telangiectasia; blackheads.

b. Rosacea.

c. The blackheads are not a feature of rosacea, although whiteheads are found in this disorder; the blackheads illustrated are found in aged skin and often co-exist with elastotic changes in the skin.

98 a. This is a scabies burrow. The adult mite can be seen as a tiny grey spot at the left-hand end of the burrow.

b. The diagnosis can be confirmed by carefully removing the mite, using a three-sided needle, and examining it under a microscope.

99 a. This is a calcified heel nodule.

b. Heel pricks made to obtain blood samples.

c. These nodules usually resolve by transepidermal elimination, after some months.

100 a. Median canaliform dystrophy (MCD). There is a well-formed split down the middle of the left thumbnail, with fir-tree-like ridges arising from it. The other thumbnail has a mild transverse nail dystrophy.

b. Nail splits in MCD resolve spontaneously, but recur. Usually only the thumbs are involved.

101 a. There is redness, swelling of the soft tissues around the nail, and proximal nail-plate dystrophy.

b. Chronic *Candida* paronychia; psoriasis; Gram-negative bacterial paronychia. Infective causes of paronychia may include: *Candida*; *Staphylococcus*; Gram-negative bacteria; herpes simplex. The involvement of several nails and associated nail dystrophy makes candida or peripheral pustular psoriasis most likely. Dermatophyte infections do not cause paronychia. If only one nail is affected, it is important to consider malignant melanoma of the nail apparatus.

102 a. Herpes simplex infection producing multiple, grouped pustules.

b. The most likely source in this instance is by way of direct inoculation during a contact sport such as rugby football – hence the term 'scrum-pox'.

103 a. Porphyria cutanea tarda (rarely, variegate porphyria).

b. Heredity; alcohol; several chlorinated benzene derivatives; oestrogen administration.

c. Specific tests for porphyrins (especially urine and faecal) and metabolites. Liver enzymes and serum iron or ferritin are usually elevated; plasma glucose may be elevated; urine is pink or may fluoresce; skin biopsy may be abnormal.

104 a. Dermatosis papularis nigra.

b. These are the small, pigmented, seborrhoeic warts that commonly appear on the faces of Afro-Caribbeans in early adult life as a normal variant. No investigation is required.

105 a. This is likely to be a pyogenic granuloma.

b. At any site, but frequently on the fingers.

c. Usually curettage or excision.

106 a. Spider naevus.

b. Solitary, or few, spider naevi are a common normal finding, especially in children. Multiple spider naevi occur in liver disease and pregnancy. The telangiectasia of systemic sclerosis do not have a central filling arteriole but fill from several different vessels.

107 a. This is atrophie blanche.
   b. Chronic venous disease, often in areas of healed ulceration.

108 a. There are multiple small dystrophic nails, with pterygium formation and nail splitting.
   b. These are features of the nail–patella syndrome, an autosomal-dominant condition.
   c. Other features are ocular (heterochromia iridis, glaucoma micro-cornea); orthopaedic (bilateral posterior iliac spines – patho-gnomonic); renal (renal dysplasia, duplicate ureters, nephrotic syndrome, glomerulonephritis).

109 a. Mongolian spot, a bluish-grey macular staining of the skin of the lumbosacral area which is common in babies of Asian or Afro-Caribbean origin. It is important not to confuse this with traumatic bruising.
   b. No investigation is required. These lesions are due to melanin in dermal melanocytes, and fade in childhood.

110 a. Paget's disease of the nipple.
   b. Atopic eczema, scabies, psoriasis (less common).
   c. These three are all likely to be bilateral, and usually sore or itchy. The absence of a palpable mass does not exclude Paget's disease.

111 a. Kerion, an inflammatory, animal-type ringworm infection.
   b. Likely to be *Trichophyton verrucosum*, from cattle.
   c. Take samples for bacteriology and mycology, then administer systemic antifungal plus antistaphylococcal antibiotic; systemic steroids may reduce inflammation and reduce risk of permanent alopecia in the beard area.

112 a. Becker's Naevus (*syn.* pigmented hairy epidermal naevus). This common condition typically appears on the chest of young men in adolescence, initially with flat pigmentation followed by the appearance of terminal hairs.
   b. It is an entirely benign type of epidermal naevus rather than due to pigment cells. It will persist.

113 a. Hidradenitis suppurativa.
  b. Simple perianal abscesses; Crohn's disease. Ordinary folliculitis is not as extensive as this.
  c. Acne, especially the severe, 'conglobate', type.

114 a. Keratoacanthoma; squamous cell carcinoma.
  b. Keratoacanthomas characteristically grow to a maximum size within approximately three months and, thereafter, resolve leaving a small, depressed scar. In the initial stages, differentiation from a rapidly growing squamous cell carcinoma may be impossible. If the clinical diagnosis is confident, the tumour can be left untreated and its size monitored to ensure that it does resolve. Alternatively the entire tumour can be treated surgically or by radiotherapy.

115 a. Thin bands of pigmentation, with a rippled appearance.
  b. Atopic eczema.
  c. It is sometimes known as 'atopic dirty neck'.

116 a. Lentigo maligna. This is a type of *in situ* melanoma in which the horizontal growth phase spreads along the basal layer of the epidermis, in contrast to the superficial spreading melanoma where malignant melanocytes spread in a haphazard fashion throughout the whole thickness of the epidermis.
  b. After 10–20 years, approximately 25% of cases develop an invasive tumour which may metastasize.

117 a. Onychogryphosis.
  b. This condition is due to neglected foot care, often with age-related thickening of the toenails.

118 a. Fish tank granuloma, caused by infection through damaged skin with *Mycobacterium marinum*. In temperate climates, the organism is commonly present in recirculated, heated water such as swimming pools or tropical fish tanks.
  b. Treatment with either cotrimoxazole, tetracycline or rifampicin for six weeks is usually curative.

119 a. Dermatitis herpetiformis. Usual sites are scalp, scapulae, sacrum, knees, elbows.
  b. Associated gluten-sensitive enteropathy.
  c. Dapsone; haemolysis and agranulocytosis.

120 a. Idiopathic systemic amyloidosis. Skin features occur in approximately 30% of patients with this condition, in contrast to secondary systemic amyloidosis due to chronic infection, where skin signs are rare. Purpuric lesions occurring in apparently normal skin after minimal trauma are characteristic of amyloidosis, and are caused by loss of vessel support due to amyloid deposition around blood vessels.

    b. When amyloid deposits become clinically obvious they appear as waxy papules, nodules or diffuse skin induration. Blisters may occur and tongue enlargement is common.

121 a. Leucocytoclastic vasculitis (*syn.* allergic vasculitis; immune complex vasculitis; Henoch–Schönlein purpura).

    b. Causes include: drug reactions (penicillin, sulphonamides, penicillamine); infections (streptococcal, hepatitis); auto-immune conditions (rheumatoid disease, systemic lupus erythematosus); protein abnormality (cryoglobulinaemia, etc.).

122 a. This is known as talon noire.

    b. Friction, causing small haemorrhages.

    c. Malignant melanoma.

123 a. Vaccination.

    b. Aluminium, present in vaccines adsorbed into aluminium hydroxide or phosphate, can cause granulomas.

    c. Where possible, use non-adsorbed vaccines; use the buttock rather than the more visible upper arm to perform vaccinations.

124 a. Onycholysis; salmon patch on the nail bed; pitting; longitudinal ridging (non-specific).

    b. Common causes of onycholysis include: skin disease (psoriasis, eczema); trauma (chemical and physical); infective (fungal, viral); systemic (thyrotoxicosis, pregnancy); drug-induced (photo-onycholysis – tetracycline, benoxaprofen); idiopathic. The combination of a salmon patch (a pinkish-brown-coloured nail bed at the proximal margin of onycholysis), pitting and onycholysis indicates psoriasis in this instance.

125 a. An irregularly shaped and pigmented plaque with eccentrically situated, darker and ulcerated, nodule.

    b. Superficial spreading melanoma, with nodular component.

126 a. Naevus sebaceous. This malformation is made up of sebaceous glands (hence the colour), apocrine glands, abnormal follicular tissue, and hyperplastic epidermis.

   b. Spontaneous resolution does not occur. At puberty, lesions become raised and lumpy. The involved area occupies the same proportion of the scalp relative to the child's head growth with age. Approximately 20% of lesions develop a basal-cell carcinoma within them in adult life.

127 a. There is an irregular linear, violaceous and pigmented band.

   b. Lichen planus, demonstrating Koebner's phenomenon.

   c. Pruritus.

128 a. The combination of broken hairs, scale and lack of scarring make a diagnosis of tinea capitis (ringworm of the scalp) most likely. Alopecia areata is unlikely because of the large amount of associated scale. Ultraviolet light examination in a darkened room may demonstrate fluorescence of individual hairs in cases of *Microsporum audouinii* and *M. canis* infections, but not in all hair fungal infections; negative findings do not exclude the diagnosis.

   b. Microscopic examination of affected hairs or scale in potassium hydroxide may reveal fungal hyphae, and fungal cultures of plucked hairs will give a definitive diagnosis.

129 a. Yellow colour, increased longitudinal curvature.

   b. Yellow nail syndrome.

   c. The syndrome is usually associated with chronic bronchitis or bronchiectasis.

130 a. This is an auricle appendage. These may be bilateral and contain skin, cartilage and fat.

   b. They are usually only cosmetic blemishes, but may be associated with more extensive and obvious developmental anomalies of the first branchial arch (e.g. Treacher–Collins syndrome).

131 a. Yes; the rash may commence several days after a typical 7-day course.

   b. Viral exanthem.

   c. A diagnostic 'challenge' would not normally be performed. However, rashes occur more frequently after ampicillin than after penicillin V, especially if administered in the context of a viral infection (95% of patients with infectious mononucleosis will develop rash if given ampicillin). A previous delayed ampicillin rash is not an absolute contraindication to the use of more basic penicillins if there is a specific indication for these; by contrast, an immediate anaphylactic or urticarial reaction would be expected to recur and is a contraindication to such therapy.

132 a. There is unilateral fine scaling of the skin on the left palm – most noticeable in the skin creases. The unilateral nature of the rash makes a fungal infection most likely and the fine white scale affecting the skin creases is characteristic of that seen in *Trichophyton rubrum* infections of the skin. Eczema, contact allergic dermatitis or psoriasis are usually symmetrical.
   b. His feet should be examined for evidence of tinea pedis.
   c. The diagnosis could be confirmed immediately by microscopic examination of skin scrapings dissolved in potassium hydroxide, and after a few weeks by fungal cultures of skin scrapings.

133 a. Acute photosensitivy (likely to be drug-induced); contact dermatitis due to an airborne allergen.
   b. This was photosensitivity due to carbamazepine (a rare cause). Other drugs which cause photosensitivity are thiazides, oral hypoglycaemics, non-steroidal anti-inflammatory drugs (NSAIDs), antibiotics (sulphonamides, tetracyclines), phenothiazines.

134 a. These are varicella blisters. There are several solitary blisters arising on patches of pink skin. Over the space of three to four days they will become haemorrhagic and then necrotic.
   b. Maternal chicken pox in early pregnancy may cause severe foetal damage resulting in central nervous system and ocular defects. Abortion may occur. If the mother develops varicella or zoster a few days before or after delivery, the neonate will have no maternal antibody and will be at risk from severe varicella, which carries a mortality of 30% if untreated.

135 a. Herpes simplex infection, transferred to the thumb in the course of sucking it.
   b. Herpetic whitlow.
   c. Staphylococcal acute paronychia and facial impetigo is possible, but would be an unusual combination.

136 a. Tuberous sclerosis: the lesions illustrated are unusually large telangiectactic papules of adenoma sebaceum.
   b. Ash leaf macules (de-pigmented macules which also arise in the scalp, producing white patches of hair called poliosis), shagreen patches (connective tissue naevi), café-au-lait spots and peri-ungual fibroma (Koenen's tumours).

137 a. Cutaneous horn (N.B. this is a description, not a diagnosis).
    b. Squamous-cell carcinoma; actinic keratosis; keratoacanthoma; seborrhoeic keratosis (the condition illustrated); viral wart.

138 a. The posterior nail fold capillaries are dilated, with several giant capillary loops, and there are segments without capillaries.
    b. Dermatomyositis. Abnormal nail fold capillaries also occur in systemic lupus erythematosus, scleroderma and long-standing Raynaud's disease.

139 a. These naevi are larger, and much more numerous, than is average for this site.
    b. Atypical naevus syndrome (dysplastic naevus syndrome, B–K mole syndrome, and several other names, may also be applied).
    c. There is an increased risk of malignant melanoma, especially in the case of a positive family history.

140 a. Eruptive xanthoma.
    b. A lipid profile showed a triglyceride of 33.3 (normal range = 0.45–1.8) mmol/l and cholesterol of 12.5 (normal range is less than 5.2) mmol/l. Lipoprotein electrophoresis revealed that this was a type I Frederickson hyperlipaemia. The patient had a strong family history of ischaemic heart disease.

141 a. A linear row of blisters on a streaky, erythematous, background.
    b. Plant-induced contact or photocontact dermatitis.
    c. Streaky pigmentation, if a photosensitizing plant was the cause (see case 64).

142 a. Cellulitis.
    b. This streptococcal infection of the dermal and subcutaneous tissues is best treated by intravenous benzyl penicillin. Associated *Staphylococcus aureus* infection may require the addition of flucloxacillin. Oral amoxycillin or cephuroxime are effective in mild cases.

143 a. This is dermatitis artefacta.

144 a. There is pronounced swelling of the soft tissues of the lip, with little surface change.
    b. Oro-facial granulomatosis, sarcoidosis, Crohn's disease, and (rarely) allergic reactions to foodstuffs, toothpaste, etc. After injury, foreign body granuloma or atypical mycobacterial infection should also be

considered. Angioedema can be excluded because it only lasts for 1–2 days. In this child a diagnosis of orofacial granulomatosis was made, and the lip settled after intralesional steroid injections.

145 a. Striate or punctate leukonychia.
   b. None; this condition was previously thought to be due to calcium deficiency, but is probably due to minor trauma.

146 a. There is redness and scaling, with post-inflammatory pigmentation, on the trunk and breast. The striking abnormality is sparing of the abdominal skin crease folds, under the breast and the right arm. In a relaxed, reclining posture, these are light-protected sites. This patient has developed very severe sunburn.
   b. Ultraviolet light effects may be enhanced by topical or systemic photosensitizers. Topical photosensitizers include: perfumed items, e.g. sunscreens, moisturizers containing bergamot; different plant species, e.g. Giant Hogweed (see case 64). Systemic photosensitizers are chiefly drugs. They include thiazides, quinine, oral hypo-glycaemics, non-steroidal anti-inflammatory agents, chlordiaz-epoxide, phenothiazines and tetracyclines.

147 a. This is likely to be molluscum contagiosum.
   b. There are discrete papular lesions with central umbilication and grouped pattern.
   c. Spontaneous resolution after 6–12 months, sometimes preceded by an itchy phase, surrounding eczema, or inflamed lesions.

148 a. Squamous-cell carcinoma (SCC) of the lip.
   b. SCCs of the lip metastasize in approximately 10% of cases.
   c. Curative treatment includes excision or radiotherapy. Alternative destructive therapies such as cryotherapy or curettage would not be appropriate in a large, invasive tumour like this.

149 a. Confluent yellowish papules in a 'cobblestoned' pattern.
   b. Pseudoxanthoma elasticum.
   c. There may be rupture of blood vessels of the retina, heart or gastrointestinal tract.

150 a. Erythema multiforme of Stevens–Johnson type.
   b. Infections (especially Herpes simplex, infectious mononucleosis, orf, mycoplasma); drugs (especially sulphonamides and other anti-biotics, anticonvulsants).

c. Whilst this example was probably triggered by Herpes simplex, oral involvement to this extent usually only occurs as a single episode (primary herpetic gingivostomatitis), and erosions at other sites would not be a likely feature.

151 a. This is erythema ab igne. Repeated heat damage produces maximal damage at the watershed areas of skin perfusion between adjacent arterioles. This results in reticulate telangiectasia, and pigmentation and hyperkeratosis following the physiological vascular mottling pattern commonly seen on the limbs (see case 21).
   b. Epidermal dysplasia and epithelioma may occur.

152 a. Oral lichenoid reaction, adjacent to an amalgam-filled tooth.
   b. Patch tests to ammoniated mercury are positive in 20% of cases, and most of these patients will improve when the amalgam is removed.

153 a. The example shown here is due to repetitive picking as a 'habit tic'.
   b. Treatment consists of explanation of the mechanism involved, to discourage the habit. Nail lacquers may hide the appearance; they may also make it less easy mechanically to damage the nail.

154 a. There are several eroded areas on her central chest and a small, flaccid blister is just visible between her breasts. The erosions are due to rapid rupture of the fragile (i.e. probably intraepidermal) blisters.
   b. This is characteristic of penicillamine-induced pemphigus erythematosus. Biopsy of a blister showed a split high in the epidermis and immunofluorescence of the clinically normal skin showed intercellular deposits of immunoglobulin G within the epidermis.

155 a. This is an example of bathing trunk naevus.
   b. Cosmetic; increased risk of malignant melanoma; occasional reports of underlying bony defects, including spina bifida occulta.

156 a. Polymorphic eruption of pregnancy (*syn.* pruritic urticarial papules and plaques of pregnancy – PUPPP). This is common in first pregnancies, and characteristically appears in the abdominal striae in the last two weeks of pregnancy. It disappears spontaneously after delivery.
   b. There is no risk to the foetus.

157 a. It is likely to be a lymph node.
   b. Secondary infection of the eczema (an area of crusting is visible).

   c. Send bacteriology swabs; apply topical steroid; administer systemic antistaphylococcal antibiotic.

158 a. The edge of the lesion is irregular, with a raised, thread-like margin. The lesion itself is depressed centrally, scaly and atrophic.

   b. Superficial basa-cell carcinoma.

159 a. Yellowish-coloured, thickened, matted hair.

   b. Confusingly called Trichomycosis axillaris, the condition is actually due to *Corynebacteria*.

   c. Usually it is sufficient to shave the hair, followed by regular washing and deodorant use.

160 a. Mycosis fungoides (cutaneous T-cell lymphoma).

   b. Before the appearance of plaques and infiltrated tumours, most patients with mycosis fungoides have a prolonged 'pre-mycotic' period in which the rash is limited to fixed, scaly, erythematous and slightly pigmented patches that may be confused with eczema or psoriasis. Many patients do not progress beyond this stage. Therapy with PUVA, retinoids and topical mustine may all produce temporary resolution and allow the patient to lead a normal life. Systemic chemotherapy is not curative.

161 a. This is likely to be caused by a contact allergy to a rubber chemical in the elasticated part of the stocking.

   b. Patch tests should be undertaken to establish the probable allergen.

162 a. These are due to a lichenoid allergic reaction to mercury salts.

   b. The reaction may slowly resolve spontaneously, although excision of the affected areas is the most effective treatment.

163 a. This type of scar is known as a keloid.

   b. Recurrence (prevented in this case by repeated intralesional steroid injections, post-operatively for six weeks).

   c. Use the buttock rather than the arm as a vaccination site, to avoid visible keloids.

164 a. Staphylococcal bullous impetigo. Most of the blisters have burst leaving the crusted discoid lesions. One small blister is present. Bullous impetigo is caused only by *S. aureus*. Non-bullous impetigo can be caused by either *S. aureus* or streptococcal (usually Lancefield group A) infection.

   b. The condition is highly infectious and the child should not go to school until adequately treated.

165 a. Pulp atrophy due to digital infarcts.

    b. Systemic sclerosis or sclerodactyly.

    c. Tight shiny skin, pigmentary disturbance, Raynaud's phenomenon, hair loss, ragged cuticles with abnormal vessels, paraesthesia.

166 a. This is likely to be tinea cruris.

    b. Toe webs; tinea pedis is almost invariably apparent.

    c. Examine skin scrapings by microscopy and mycological culture.

167 a. Lupus erythematosus, of systemic or subacute cutaneous type.

    b. Anti-Ro (anti-SSA) antibody; the combination of 'butterfly' malar rash with photosensitivity and negative antinuclear antibody (ANA) is strongly suggestive of subacute cutaneous lupus erythematosus (SCLE), in which anti-SSA is usually positive.

    c. Arthralgia is frequent, but other significant systemic disease rare, in SCLE.

168 a. There is marked colour variation, with reds, flesh tones (areas of spontaneous resolution), browns, blacks and greys. The edge is irregular, with notching or indentation.

    b. Superficial spreading malignant melanoma.

169 a. Dermatomyositis.

    b. Limb girdle weakness.

    c. Prove the diagnosis (by way of skin biopsy, muscle enzymes, electromyography, muscle biopsy), and search for underlying cause (underlying malignancy in at least 25% of adult cases; overlap with other autoimmune disorders).

170 a. Acrocyanosis. This is a relatively common finding in young women, characterized by cyanotic discolouration of the extremities which is made worse by cold. By comparison with Raynaud's phenomenon, which is intermittent, acrocyanosis is consistently present to some extent.

    b. Peripheral cyanosis due to cardiovascular or lung disease and hyperviscosity syndromes must be excluded.

171 a. There is heaped-up scaling with matted hairs. Removal of a piece of scale also results in removal of a small bunch of hair.

    b. This is pityriasis amiantacea (*syn.* tinea amiantacea), so called because it was considered to look like asbestos ore. It is a type of scalp eczema. Scalp psoriasis can produce a similar picture.

172 a. This is an allergy to the adhesive tape used to secure an intravenous cannula.
b. Patch tests may prove allergy to colophony or other adhesive resins.

173 a. Acneiform drug eruption; folliculitis; eruptive xanthoma.
b. Acneiform drug eruptions are caused by: hormones (corticosteroids, androgens); antituberculous therapy (ethambutol, isoniazid, rifampicin); halogens (iodine, bromides and chlorinated hydrocarbons); anticonvulsants (phenytoin); others (frusemide, lithium, doxycyclin).
c. The pustules all have the same morphology, unlike in acne vulgaris, where lesions including comedones, papules and pustules are all present in the same patient.

174 a. Alopecia in male pattern (bi-temporal recession).
b. Androgenic hormone-secreting tumour, usually ovarian.
c. Pelvic examination, ultrasound of abdomen, biochemical androgen screen.

175 a. The history and distribution of the blisters suggest that they have been produced as a result of minimal frictional forces. This suggests epidermolysis bullosa (EB).
b. There are many types of EB, with widely differing prognoses. An appropriate biopsy should be taken for immunofluorescence and electron microscopy, to determine the type and hence the prognosis.
c. Other causes of perinatal blistering that should also be considered include: staphylococcal scalded skin syndrome, which produces skin shedding rather than blisters; accidental burns, although the symmetrical distribution and widespread involvement here make this improbable in this child.

176 a. They are striae due to rapid vertical growth.
b. They may be confused with whipmarks, or with striae due to Cushing's syndrome.
c. They will persist, but become white rather than pink in colour

177 a. Palmar psoriasis.
b. Dermatitis; fungal infection.
c. Relative lack of symptoms makes dermatitis unlikely; symmetry makes fungal infection unlikely; sharp demarcation is typical of psoriasis.

178 a. Pityriasis rosea. This is suggested by the characteristic, oval-shaped, erythematous plaques with central clearing which occur on the trunk and proximal limbs.

    b. The patient should be asked about a possible herald patch, i.e. a solitary plaque, now bigger than the rest, that appeared a few days before the rash became more widespread.

    c. The two differential diagnoses not to be missed are a drug eruption, and secondary syphilis – the latter is not usually itchy and mucus membrane lesions occur. Tinea corporis is excluded by the symmetrical distribution.

179 a. Subungual haematoma.

    b. No pigmentation of the nail fold or adjacent skin; red and blue-black colour rather than brown pigment; smaller haematoma under second toenail; short history.

180 a. Pyoderma gangrenosum. Note the typical blue, inflammatory edge.

    b. Inflammatory bowel disease; myeloproliferative disorders; inflammatory arthritides.

    c. Cyclosporin.

181 a. Look for scalp changes suggestive of fungal infection (scaling, redness, broken hairs) or collagen vascular disease (scarring alopecia). Inherited hair shaft abnormalities are unlikely to present for the first time in adult life. Broken (indicative of trichotillomania, alopecia areata, fungal infections) and 'exclamation mark' (alopecia areata) hairs must be looked for.

    b. Causes of gradual diffuse hair loss include: myxoedema; hyperthyroidism; iron deficiency; drugs (anticoagulants, anticonvulsants, carbimazole); idiopathic diffuse hair loss; androgenic alopecia; diffuse pattern alopecia areata.

    c. A ferritin and thyroid stimulating hormone level are essential. In the absence of supporting physical signs or symptoms, further tests are unnecessary.

182 a. Scattered blue-black punctate spots (a few yellow papules of an eruptive xanthoma are also present).

    b. Carbon deposits in the skin.

    c. This is a 'blast tattoo' acquired whilst mining coal.

183 a. Juvenile forefoot dermatosis; contact allergic eczema; tinea pedis; eczema.

    b. Juvenile forefoot dermatosis is a common dermatitis of the foot seen in prepubertal children. It is due to frictional damage to the skin leading to reduced sweating. Paradoxically the frictional damage appears to occur initially because of increased foot sweating produced by impervious footwear.

184 a. There is a patch of hair thinning, with multiple short hairs, on the crown of her head, with a well-defined border.

b. When broken hairs are present, alopecia areata, fungal infection and trichotillomania must all be considered. The diagnosis of tricho-tillomania or hair pulling is suggested by the presence of multiple broken anagen hairs that cannot be plucked easily; remaining hairs are usually less than 3mm long because it is difficult to pull out shorter hairs. When viewed through a microscope, these have a broken-off end rather than a dystrophic, 'exclamation mark', appearance. Fungal infections have associated scale and inflammation.

185 a. Toxic epidermal necrolysis.

b. Antibiotics (penicillin, tetracyclines, sulphonamides); anticonvuls-ants (especially phenytoin and barbiturates); allopurinol, butazones.

c. Conjunctivae and cilia may be lost with subsequent scarring, leading to symblepharon, ectropion or entropion, and corneal opacities.

186 a. There are multiple lesions on the sole of the big toe, with super-ficially punched-out areas.

b. Pitted keratolysis, due to a keratin infection with *Corynebacteria*. It usually occurs as a result of increased foot sweating. Bacterial enzymes produce the keratolysis, giving rise to the characteristic smell.

c. Treatment involves reducing sweating and destroying the bacteria with topical antibiotics, e.g. mupirocin ointment.

187 a. Inframammary intertrigo.

b. Both are due to candidiasis.

c. Satellite lesions suggest the diagnosis of candidiasis.

188 a. Dermographism. (Dermatologists would not normally elicit weals unnecessarily; this patient volunteered to have her dramatic condition photographed.)

b. Physical urticaria.

c. The vast majority of cases have no identifiable cause.

189 a. The lesions have an inward-pointing keratotic rim with a central depression or scarred area.

b. Disseminated superficial actinic porokeratosis. This is a relatively common disorder, usually seen on areas exposed to the sun, especially the lower leg and forearm of middle-aged women. It may coexist with actinic keratoses.

190 a. The lesion is likely to be a dental sinus.
   b. Orthopantogram, to identify the underlying site of infection; bacteriology cultures, if any discharge can be identified.

191 a. Port wine stain (capillary naevus).
   b. These are flat in childhood but frequently become nodular in adult life. Malignant transformation is not a recognized complication.
   c. Laser treatment, either flash-lamp pumped pulsed dye or argon-pumped tuneable dye, is the current best therapy.

192 a. There is poorly defined pitting with a rather rippled appearance; loss of cuticles; shiny nail surface.
   b. Eczema/dermatitis; the pits are less sharply defined than those typical of psoriasis, and there are no other nail changes of this disorder; the shiny nail surface is a feature of rubbing itchy skin.
   c. Psoriasis; alopecia areata.

193 a. Hereditary haemorrhagic telangiectasia (Osler–Rendu–Weber disease).
   b. History of other affected family members (autosomal-dominant); recurrent nose bleeds; symptoms of anaemia.
   c. Other features include telangiectasia at all other skin and mucosal sites, especially the tongue, lips, fingers, nail beds and conjunctiva. Arteriovenous malformations with shunting may occur in the lungs (producing cyanosis and clubbing) and liver.

194 a. This is likely to be Bowen's disease.
   b. Psoriasis.
   c. Previous (probably childhood) exposure to arsenic in a 'tonic'.

195 a. Minoxidil, cyclosporin, phenytoin, androgenic steroids, progestogens.
   b. Male pattern scalp hair loss, breast atrophy, clitoral enlargement, recent development of terminal hair in male sexual pattern sites.

196 a. Tuberous sclerosis with shagreen patch ('cobblestoned' patch of rough skin) and three flat ash-leaf macules.
   b. Ash-leaf macules can be detected using Wood's light examination in a darkened room; as these are usually the first sign of this disorder, this test should be performed in all potentially affected children.

197 a. Plaque psoriasis. The central plaque has been gently scraped and shows the white, scaly surface more clearly than the surrounding plaques.

b. Topical treatments include: emollients, keratolytics (e.g. salicylic acid), tar, dithranol, topical steroids and vitamin D analogues.

198 a. This is a 'nit', the egg case of the common head louse. An adult female louse attaches 150–300 eggs to the base of hair shafts. The larva hatches out one week later, leaving the empty egg case firmly glued onto the hair. This grows out with the hair. The larva moults three times and reaches sexual maturity in three weeks.

b. Topical malathion, carbaryl or pyrethroids.

199 a. There is thinning of the cheek skin, with pronounced telangiectasia. This is characteristic of corticosteroid-induced collagen atrophy of the skin.

b. These changes are irreversible.

200 a. Palmoplantar pustulosis (localized pustular psoriasis).

b. Tinea pedis.

c. This disorder is strongly associated with cigarette smoking. Alcohol history may be important if systemic therapy is indicated; occupation and social circumstances are relevant as this can be a chronic and disabling condition.

INDEX